795

COMBATTING CARDIOVASCULAR DISEASES SKILLFULLY

COMBATTING CARDIOVASCULAR DISEASES SKILLFULLY

Nursing78 Books
Intermed Communications, Inc.
Horsham, Pennsylvania

NURSING78 BOOKS

PUBLISHER: Eugene W. Jackson
Editorial Director: Daniel L. Cheney
Clinical Director: Margaret Van Meter, RN
Graphics Director: John Isely
Business Manager: Tom Temple

NURSING SKILLBOOK SERIES
Editorial staff for this volume:
Book Editor: Helen Hamilton
Clinical Editors: Minnie Rose, RN, BSN, MEd, Catherine Manzi, RN
Marginalia Editor: Avery Rome
Copy Editor: Patricia Hamilton
Researcher and Indexer: Vonda Heller
Production Manager: Bernard Haas
Typography Manager: David C. Kosten
Production Assistant: Betty Mancini
Designer: Maggie Arnott
Artists: Robert Goldstein, Robert Jackson, Robert Renn, Sandra Simms
Cover and Divider Art: Robert Goldstein

Clinical Consultants

Kathleen Dracup, BSN, MN, *Clinical Professor, University of California at Los Angeles School of Nursing, Los Angeles, Calif.*
Peter G. Lavine, MD, *Director of Coronary Care Unit, Crozer-Chester Medical Center, Chester, Pa.*
Despina Seremelis, RN, BSN, *Staff Nurse, Temple University Hospital, Philadelphia, Pa.*

Copyright © 1974, 1975, 1977, 1978
by Intermed Communications, Inc.
132 Welsh Road, Horsham, Pa. 19044
All rights reserved. Reproduction in whole or
part by any means whatsoever without written
permission of the publisher is prohibited by law.

Library of Congress Cataloging in Publication Data
Main entry under title:

COMBATTING CARDIOVASCULAR DISEASES SKILLFULLY

"Nursing Skillbook series."
Bibliography: p. 191
Includes index.
1. Cardiovascular disease nursing. [DNLM: 1. Cardiovascular diseases — Nursing. WY152.5 C729]
RC674.C63   610.73'6   78-21667
ISBN 0-916730-11-5

CONTENTS

Foreword 9
Rose Pinneo, RN, MS

In children: Recognize congenital abnormalities
1. Cardiovascular assessment: Know the norms 15
   By Marie Scott Brown, RN, PhD and
   Mary Alexander Murphy, RN, MSN
2. Cardiac babies: Know six common anomalies 23
   By Kathy Murphy, RN, BSN, MSN and
   Kit Stahler, RN, BSN, MSN
3. Cardiac surgery: Know how to cope 33
   By Kit Stahler, RN, BSN, MSN and
   Kathy Murphy, RN, BSN, MSN
Skillcheck 1 41

In adults: Deal with acquired disease
4. Assessment: Review of vital skills 45
   By Christine Sue Breu, RN, BSN, MN
5. Diagnostic tests: Invasive and noninvasive 55
   By Arlene B. Strong, RN, MN
6. Hypertension: Risk factor in atherosclerosis 67
   By Rosemary Jarlath Maloney, BSN, MSN
7. Coronary artery disease: Stages of progression 75
   By Christine W. Cannon, RN, MSN
8. Acute myocardial infarction: Severe ASHD 83
   By Catherine Ciaverelli Manzi, RN
9. Congestive failure: Severe cardiac impairment 93
   By Lauren Marie Isacson, RN and
   Klaus J. Schulz, MD
10. Cardiac complications: Often catastrophic 103
    By Sally A. Bowers, RN
11. Inflammatory heart diseases: Four most common .115
    By Mary M. Canobbio, RN, BSN
12. Cardiomyopathy: Mysterious dysfunction 125
    By Kathleen A. Dracup, RN, MN
13. Pulmonary embolism: Hazard of immobilization . .133
    By M. Sandy Wyper, RN, MSN

14. Pacemakers: Help for the faltering heart 141
    By Minnie Bowen Rose, RN, BSN, MEd
Skillcheck 2 151

In the elderly: Expect vascular deterioration
15. Peripheral vascular disease: Cause of leg pain 155
    By Idabelle Ream, RN
16. Aneurysm: Potentially fatal defect 163
    By Gail D'Onofrio Long, RN, MS
Skillcheck 3 169

Skillcheck answers 171

Appendices
Cardiac rehabilitation plan for graduated
activity and exercise 173

Some heart-saving advice for patients
after discharge 174

Emergency cardiovascular drugs 175

Glossary 179

Common cardiovascular abbreviations 184

Index 185

Suggested further reading 191

AUTHORS

Sally A. Bowers, a graduate of Johns Hopkins Hospital School of Nursing, is a staff nurse in the cardiovascular intensive care unit, Toronto Western Hospital, Canada. She completed a training program in coronary care at the University of Maryland, Baltimore.

Christine Sue Breu received her BSN from Marian College of Fond du Lac in Michigan. She earned her MN from the University of California at Los Angeles School of Nursing where she is now a cardiovascular nurse specialist in the University Hospital.

Marie Scott Brown is an associate professor of parent-child nursing at the University of Colorado School of Nursing where she received her MSN, MA, and PhD. She is a BSN graduate of Marquette University, Milwaukee, Wisconsin. She is a member of the National Association for Pediatric Nurse Associates and Practitioners.

Christine W. Cannon holds a BS from the University of Pennsylvania, Philadelphia. She is a medical clinical specialist at Wilmington Medical Center. She belongs to the American Association of Critical Care Nurses and Sigma Theta Tau.

Mary M. Canobbio is a nurse-teacher-practitioner at Kaiser Permanente Medical Center, Los Angeles. An AA graduate of Los Angeles City College, Department of Nursing, she earned her BSN at California State University (L.A.). She's working towards an MN.

Kathleen A. Dracup, an advisor on this book, is an assistant clinical professor at the University of California at Los Angeles School of Nursing where she also received her MN. Her BSN is from St. Xavier's College, Chicago.

Lauren Marie Isacson graduated from the Ann May School of Nursing, Jersey Shore Medical Center, Neptune, New Jersey, where she is an inservice instructor. She is a student at Trenton State University.

Gail D'Onofrio Long received her BS from Duke University, Durham, North Carolina, and her MS from Boston University where she is a clinical specialist in the medical intensive/coronary care units. She holds a certificate in advanced life support.

Rosemary Jarlath Maloney is a clinical nurse at Tripler Army Medical Center, Honolulu, Hawaii. She is a BSN graduate of Gwynedd Mercy College, Springhouse, Pennsylvania, and an MSN graduate of the University of Pennsylvania.

Catherine Ciaverelli Manzi graduated from Hahnemann Hospital School of Nursing where she was formerly head nurse of the cardiac intensive care center. She is presently a clinical editor for the Nursing Skillbook series and a student at Holy Family College.

Kathy Murphy is an instructor at the University of Pennsylvania School of Nursing where she received her MSN. She received her BSN from the University of Maine, Portland. She is a member of the American Association of Critical Care Nurses.

Mary Alexander Murphy received her BSN, MS, and nurse practitioner certification from the University of Colorado, Denver, where she is an instructor in the school of medicine, department of pediatrics. She is a doctoral candidate at the University of Denver.

Idabelle Ream is a diploma graduate of Philadelphia General Hospital. She is patient care coordinator, critical care service, at Hahnemann Medical College and Hospital, Philadelphia, and is a member of the American Association of Critical Care Nurses.

Minnie Bowen Rose received her BSN from Indiana University, Bloomington, Indiana, and her MEd from Temple University, Philadelphia. She is a clinical editor for the Nursing Skillbook series.

Klaus J. Schulz is a director of the cardiovascular laboratory and pacemaker evaluation center at Jersey Shore Medical Center, Neptune, New Jersey. He attended medical school in Berlin, Germany.

Kit Stahler has recently completed her education, taking her BSN and MSN from the University of Pennsylvania. She is a member of the American Association of Critical Care Nurses, and of the National Association of Pediatric Nurses Associates and Practitioners.

Arlene B. Strong is a cardiac clinical specialist at the V.A. Hospital, Portland, Oregon. Her BSN was acquired at the University of Portland, and her MN at the University of Oregon, Portland. She is a member of the American Council on Cardiovascular Nursing.

M. Sandy Wyper received her BSN and MSN from Case Western Reserve University, Cleveland, Ohio, where she teaches medical-surgical nursing at Frances Payne Bolton School of Nursing. She holds membership in the honor society, Sigma Theta Tau.

FOREWORD

Cardiovascular nursing no longer means just the care of patients in the coronary care unit. Besides direct nursing care, nurses are expected to promote health and prevent cardiovascular disease in many ways.

Technological advances in diagnosis and treatment...sophisticated equipment available for patient support...current trends toward early detection and prevention of risk factors...and increased emphasis on rehabilitation and patient teaching...all have greatly expanded nurses' responsibilities to patients with cardiovascular disease. What are some of these expanded responsibilities? For example, nurses now screen patients for blood pressure abnormalities and give counseling about this and other risk factors. General staff nurses are usually responsible for preparing the cardiac patient for discharge through teaching and discharge planning. And, public health nurses run community clinics designed to help people who need supervision during chronic illness. These clinics offer help with long-term management of hypertension, congestive heart failure, and pacemakers.

To participate in health care in these important ways, you must have highly developed skills in physical assessment, history taking, diagnostic test interpretation and health teaching. Your contribution via nursing assessment can hardly be overstated. Although you don't establish the patient's diagnosis of cardiovascular disease, you must oversee his progress under treatment. No patient's condition remains static. In case of serious cardiovascular disease, improvement means a chance for survival; deterioration can mean sudden death. Unquestionably then, every patient with cardiovascular disease needs continuing assessment of his physiological status and of his response to treatment. Such assessment is primarily a nursing task, and the skills and enthusiasm you bring to this task profoundly influence the patient's survival.

This Skillbook can help you review and update the skills you need to offer patients with cardiovascular disease the best possible care. The book begins with a brief review of pediatric cardiology (which includes congenital anomalies and their surgical correction). It continues with the most common forms of acquired cardiovascular disease in adults. This, the most comprehensive section of the book, includes: a detailed review of physical assessment in adults; a summary of the most useful diagnostic studies (which tells how nurses can prepare patients for these tests and how to understand their results); and, in several chapters, a discussion of coronary artery disease in its various stages of severity. The same section includes chapters that tell how to recognize and deal with cardiomyopathy (a little known condition) and inflammatory diseases of the heart. Other chapters in this section tell how to cope with cardiogenic shock, pulmonary edema, and pacemakers. The final section of this book deals briefly with the management of vascular disease including peripheral vascular disease and aneurysms.

Throughout, this book focuses on the nurse's role as a member of the health team. It tells what symptoms to expect and how to evaluate them; how to recognize important complications; how to plan, coordinate, and provide total care; how to provide psychological support; and, how to help with rehabilitation. A nurse who does all of these things well can help restore the patient to his maximal potential.

All in all, this book offers a handy reference to cardiovascular nursing. Mastering its contents can help you to improve your care of patients with cardiovascular disease and make you a more valuable member of the health care team. The resulting confidence in the quality of care you feel competent to give can only enhance your satisfaction in nursing.

—ROSE PINNEO, RN, MS
Associate Professor of Nursing
University of Rochester
Rochester, N.Y.

IN CHILDREN:

OGNIZE CONGENITAL ABNORMALITIES

1

Cardiovascular Assessment
Know the norms

BY MARIE SCOTT BROWN, RN, PhD and
MARY ALEXANDER MURPHY, RN, MSN

OBVIOUSLY, MOST CHILDREN have no cardiovascular problems at all. But the unlucky ones who do are always seriously — and often fatally — ill.

Children's cardiovascular problems stem from congenital heart disease or from rheumatic fever. Congenital heart disease is the leading cause of serious illness and death in babies and newborns; rheumatic fever, the second largest cause of cardiac problems in children over age five. Even if you don't specialize in the care of children, you should know how to recognize children with these potentially fatal problems. This chapter will tell you how.

First, look at the whole child
Begin by carefully looking at the whole child. His skin tones and breathing pattern can tell you a lot. Look for the common signs of heart failure: pallor, fretfulness, inability to suckle, and uneasy breathing.

Carefully check his skin and mucous membranes, for they can tell you a lot about the health of the cardiovascular system. For example, pallor in an infant often spells severe heart problems. Look for cyanosis. It will usually appear first in the

Normal respiratory rates

AGE	RATE
Birth	30-40
1st year	26-30
2nd year	20-26
Adolescence	20

lips, nailbeds, or ear lobes. Any persistent cyanosis is a matter of serious concern. Cyanosis is often associated with polycythemia (a hematocrit over 70%, usually).

Remember that mild cyanosis may be normal in an infant, but evaluate it with care. Normal cyanosis should *not:*
- be excessive or persistent
- cover the entire body, or
- be darker in the arms than in the legs.

Report any abnormal cyanosis to a doctor, for it points to cardiovascular or respiratory difficulty. Also, look for edema of any part. It is rare in newborns, but when it occurs, it tends to appear in the eyelids.

Respiratory and other symptoms

Sometimes respiratory symptoms are just that. But they can also reflect cardiovascular problems. So, with this in mind, evaluate symptoms such as dyspnea, orthopnea, and frequent upper respiratory infections. Also think of and look for cardiovascular problems when you see certain other curious symptoms in children:
- continuous squatting and sleeping in the knee-chest position; this is almost diagnostic of a cardiac problem (usually tetralogy of Fallot)
- easy fatigability in an older child; in an infant, falling asleep immediately after taking only 2 to 2½ oz of milk
- excessively labored breathing in an infant during defecation
- anorexia, vomiting, profuse sweating
- delayed growth and development, especially in an infant (failure to thrive)
- enlarged liver
- clubbing of the fingers and toes
- enlarged heart
- pulsating neck vessels
- tachypnea without retractions.

Evaluate pulse and blood pressure

Don't overlook the importance of measuring pulse and blood pressures. They are as important to the physical examination as they are commonplace. Remember, normal values change according to the child's age. So, keep handy a list of the normal values (see page 18) to help you evaluate them correctly.

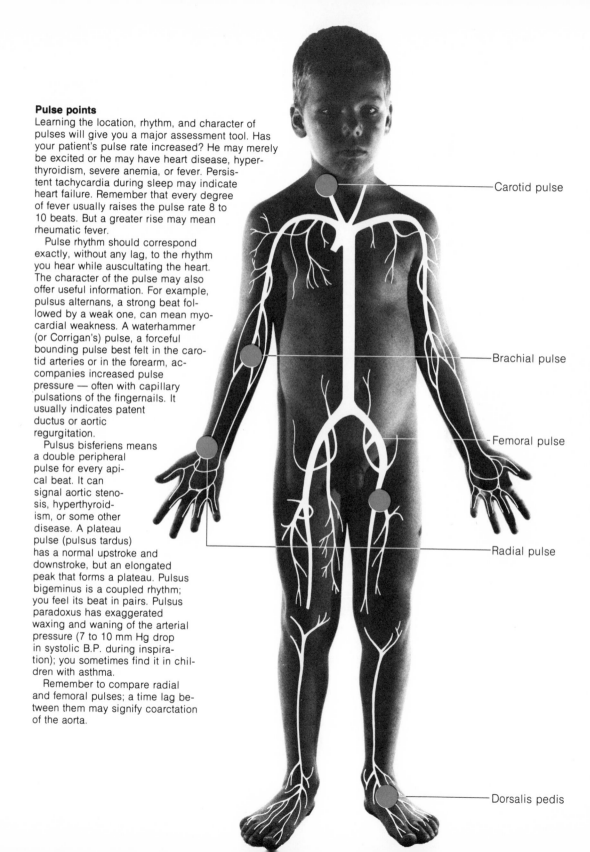

Pulse points

Learning the location, rhythm, and character of pulses will give you a major assessment tool. Has your patient's pulse rate increased? He may merely be excited or he may have heart disease, hyperthyroidism, severe anemia, or fever. Persistent tachycardia during sleep may indicate heart failure. Remember that every degree of fever usually raises the pulse rate 8 to 10 beats. But a greater rise may mean rheumatic fever.

Pulse rhythm should correspond exactly, without any lag, to the rhythm you hear while auscultating the heart. The character of the pulse may also offer useful information. For example, pulsus alternans, a strong beat followed by a weak one, can mean myocardial weakness. A waterhammer (or Corrigan's) pulse, a forceful bounding pulse best felt in the carotid arteries or in the forearm, accompanies increased pulse pressure — often with capillary pulsations of the fingernails. It usually indicates patent ductus or aortic regurgitation.

Pulsus bisferiens means a double peripheral pulse for every apical beat. It can signal aortic stenosis, hyperthyroidism, or some other disease. A plateau pulse (pulsus tardus) has a normal upstroke and downstroke, but an elongated peak that forms a plateau. Pulsus bigeminus is a coupled rhythm; you feel its beat in pairs. Pulsus paradoxus has exaggerated waxing and waning of the arterial pressure (7 to 10 mm Hg drop in systolic B.P. during inspiration); you sometimes find it in children with asthma.

Remember to compare radial and femoral pulses; a time lag between them may signify coarctation of the aorta.

Carotid pulse

Brachial pulse

Femoral pulse

Radial pulse

Dorsalis pedis

Know the norms

Newborn infants have rapid, fluctuating pulse rates that increase with activity or crying and decrease sharply during sleep. The irregular pulse rhythms of a newborn seem to be related to respiration. During childhood strong physical or emotional stimuli can drive the pulse rate up rapidly. You'll find a rate higher in the morning than in the afternoon and higher after meals than before. In adolescents you may find tachycardia normal, especially in girls; or, a pulse rate as slow as 40 per minute, often in athletic boys. Note, too, that during adolescence, girls' pulse rates are regularly higher than boys'. In any case, persistent tachycardia or hypertension should be investigated.

To measure arterial blood pressure accurately in small children, make sure the arm cuff covers no more than two-thirds and no less than one-half of the patient's upper arm. Blood pressure varies with the age, height, and weight of the child. You'll find many increases during adolescence: Excitement or activity can drive systolic pressure up to as much as 40 to 50 mm Hg above normal. Remember, too, that if the patient isn't quiet, you'll get a falsely high reading. Variation seems to be the rule, so know what is normal for your patient.

AVERAGE PULSE RATE AT REST				
AGE	NORMAL RANGE		AVERAGE	
Newborn	70-170		120	
1-11 months	80-160		120	
2 years	80-130		110	
4 years	80-120		100	
6 years	75-115		100	
8 years	70-110		90	
10 years	70-110		90	
	Girls	Boys	Girls	Boys
12 years	70-110	65-105	90	85
14 years	65-105	60-100	85	80
16 years	60-100	55-95	80	75
18 years	55-95	50-90	75	70

AVERAGE BLOOD PRESSURE AT REST		
AGE	GIRLS	BOYS
4 years	98/60	98/55
6 years	105/65	105/60
8 years	108/67	105/60
10 years	112/64	110/65
12 years	115/65	110/65
14 years	112/65	114/65

There are actually five sounds in a blood-pressure reading, but most clinicians cannot accurately hear them all. You should be able to hear and record at least three:
- the point at which you first hear the sounds
- the point at which they become muffled
- the point at which they disappear.

According to the American Heart Association, in children, the point of muffling should be considered the diastolic.

Next, examine the chest

To examine the chest itself, you can use inspection, palpation, percussion, and auscultation. Let's consider these in turn. Inspection of the chest is best done with the patient flat on his back, his rib cage elevated to 45 degrees. Tangential lighting is best. You can get the most accurate assessments at the end of each breath. Look for the point of maximal impulse (usually at the 5th intercostal space at the midclavicular line) and for abnormal lifts or heaves.

Also look for deformities in the shape of the chest that may alter the heart's position. Some of them, such as Marfan's syndrome (its primary lesion, dilatation of the aorta), are associated with heart problems. Others are not.

Percussion can help outline the borders of the heart, but is rarely used by nurses. During *palpation* and *auscultation* you examine five areas for any abnormal sounds, murmurs, or thrills — a sensation like holding a purring kitten.

Listen for heart sounds

You really have to develop your own system for auscultation. But a good way is to inch your stethoscope around all five areas of the chest, first with the bell and then with the diaphragm. Do this with the child in five positions: standing; sitting straight; sitting with the chest bent forward; lying flat on the back; and lying on the left side.

With the stethoscope, you can follow up on all the leads uncovered by earlier parts of the examination and look for new ones. The first thing to check is the normalcy of heart sounds.

When listening to heart sounds, concentrate on four characteristics: rate, intensity, and rhythm of the regular sounds (see page 20), and watch for abnormal sounds — rubs, clicks, or murmurs. Evaluate the rate as you would evaluate a peripheral pulse. The apical and radial pulse should be simultaneous, or at least without significant lag.

The normal heart sounds are S_1 (lub) and S_2 (dub). S_1 represents the sound heard at the closure of the tricuspid and mitral valves. S_2 represents closure of the aortic and pulmonic valves.

Intensity of S_1 is normally greater than that of S_2 at the apex (*lub*-dub); S_2 is normally greater at the base (lub-*dub*). Increased intensity of S_1 at the base may mean recent exercise, or even anemia, fever, or tachycardia. Decreased intensity of S_1 is usually more serious and can accompany an infarct. A loud S_1 with a slow heart rate (60 to 80, for instance) may mean mitral stenosis, heart block, or atrial flutter. An S_1 that constantly changes intensity, with a slow heart rate, may mean a heart block. Loud S_2 may be normal, or it may indicate coarctation or arterial hypertension.

Evaluate heart rhythm very carefully. Listen for irregularity; then decide whether it follows any pattern. If it does not, notify the doctor. The patient needs further evaluation with EKGs or a cardiac monitor. Remember, sinus arrhythmia is common in the young.

A common example of abnormal heart rhythm is *atrial*

Cuffs count

An accurate blood pressure reading depends on the proper cuff size. You should have cuffs in all the standard sizes — 2.5 inches, 5 inches, 8 inches, and 12 inches.

Since you can't easily hear the blood pressure in babies under a year old, use the flush technique. Make sure the baby is quiet, then elevate his arm or leg to drain blood from it. (This makes the arterial flow easier to hear.) Apply the blood pressure cuff, inflate it, and lower the baby's limb. As you deflate the cuff gradually, observe the point at which the limb distal to the cuff flushes with color. This is the mean systolic-diastolic pressure.

Taking thigh blood pressures can also provide helpful information. In infants, the systolic pressure in the thigh should equal that in the arm. In children older than one year, the systolic thigh pressure may be from 10 to 44 mm Hg higher than the arm pressure, but the diastolic should still be the same. If it's lower, suspect coarctation.

Don't overlook the pulse pressure — the difference between the systolic and the diastolic readings. Normally, this difference throughout childhood is about 20 to 50 mm Hg. If the pulse pressure is wide (more than 50), is it because of a low diastolic reading? If you're using the proper cuff size, then suspect a patent ductus arteriosus, aortic regurgitation, or other serious heart disease. With a high systolic reading, increased pulse pressure could be due to fever, excitement, or recent exercise. An abnormally *narrow* pulse pressure (less than 20) suggests aortic stenosis.

Sounds of the heart

- S₁: the systolic part of the cardiac cycle; the closing of the mitral and tricuspid valves makes this the "lub" of the "lub-dub"; loudest at the apex (5th ICS, midclavicular line).

- S₂: diastole; closure of the aortic and pulmonary valves at the end of systole; shorter and higher in pitch than S₁ and louder than S₁ at the base (2nd ICS); this is the "dub" of "lub-dub."

- S₃: rapid ventricular filling; occasionally heard if ventricular failure or valvular incompetency is present; a low-pitched, early diastolic sound (like the "y" in "Kentucky" where "Ken" and "tuck" represent S₁ and S₂) coming from blood rushing through the mitral and tricuspid valves, hitting empty ventricles. If caused by a left-sided dysfunction, it's best heard in the mitral area; if by a right-sided dysfunction, in the tricuspid area. This sound can be normal in a child but almost never in an adult.

- S₄: an audible atrial contraction at the very end of diastole; rapid filling into a ventricle with decreased compliance. Sounds like the "Ten" in "Tennessee" where "nes" and "see" represent S₁ and S₂; almost never normal, especially in children; more often heard in persons over 65; best heard at the apex.

- Summation gallop: all four heart sounds are present but S₃ and S₄ fuse because of a rapid heart rate (above 110 BPM); occurs in mid-diastole, best heard at the apex of the heart.

fibrillation. At first, this sounds very fast but regular. Listen more carefully, and you will realize that a few beats are being dropped. This is always abnormal. It can mean organic heart disease, rheumatic fever, thyrotoxicosis, or some other serious illness.

Common arrhythmias

The most common arrhythmia is sinus arrhythmia. The heart speeds up with inspiration and slows down with expiration. This arrhythmia does occur in normal children. To distinguish it from abnormal rhythms, you can ask an older child to hold his breath. If it is sinus arrhythmia, it should disappear. In an infant, you simply have to listen very closely to see if it fluctuates with respiration.

Bigeminy (coupled rhythm) consists of a normal beat followed by a premature contraction. Normal in some children, it may indicate organic heart disease in others. Premature beats, either atrial or ventricular, can be normal or not. Report all arrhythmias to a doctor.

Listen for unusual sounds

These come in a dizzying variety, not only S₃ and S₄, but rubs, crunches, clicks, snaps, splits, hums, and murmurs — each with meaning. S₃ is best heard at the apex with the bell of the stethoscope. It may be normal in a child, but sometimes it is really a gallop rhythm and pathological (it is always abnormal in an adult). S₃ is the diastolic (ventricular) sound that reflects rapid filling time of the ventricle. It is usually a sign of fluid overload or ventricular dysfunction. You can hear the S₄ best at the apex, too. In infants and children, it's much more rare than S₃, and is almost always abnormal. It can indicate aortic stenosis, hypertension, anemia, and hyperthyroidism. S₄ is the atrial sound at the end of diastole.

A pericardial friction rub is always abnormal. This is a scratchy, high-pitched, grating sound. It may or may not be affected by respiration. What distinguishes it from the quite similar pleural rub: The pericardial friction rub lasts only a few days; the pleural rub, much longer. Also, the pericardial friction rub extends through both systole and diastole, and you can hear it best when the patient leans forward and exhales deeply.

Hammon's sign, a mediastinal crunch, is a randomly dis-

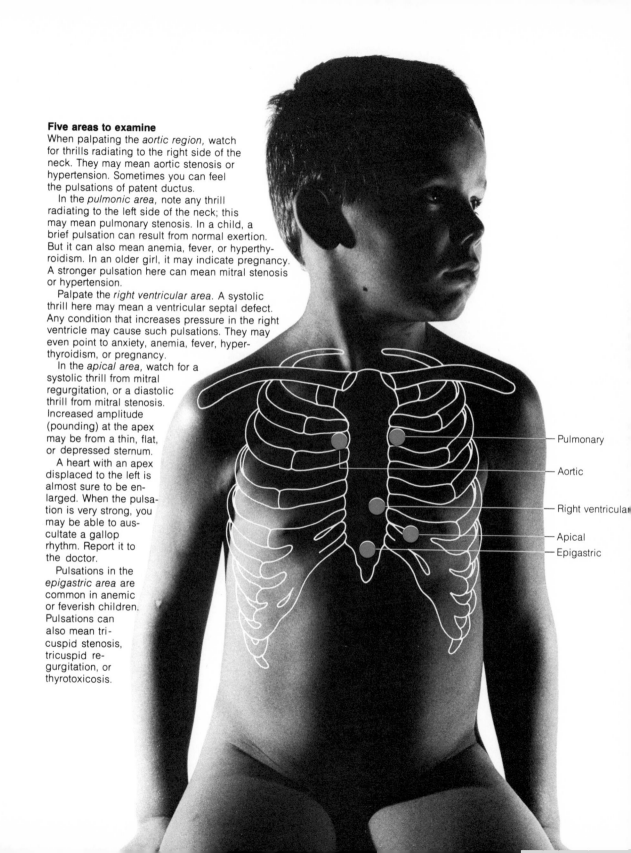

Five areas to examine

When palpating the *aortic region,* watch for thrills radiating to the right side of the neck. They may mean aortic stenosis or hypertension. Sometimes you can feel the pulsations of patent ductus.

In the *pulmonic area,* note any thrill radiating to the left side of the neck; this may mean pulmonary stenosis. In a child, a brief pulsation can result from normal exertion. But it can also mean anemia, fever, or hyperthyroidism. In an older girl, it may indicate pregnancy. A stronger pulsation here can mean mitral stenosis or hypertension.

Palpate the *right ventricular area.* A systolic thrill here may mean a ventricular septal defect. Any condition that increases pressure in the right ventricle may cause such pulsations. They may even point to anxiety, anemia, fever, hyperthyroidism, or pregnancy.

In the *apical area,* watch for a systolic thrill from mitral regurgitation, or a diastolic thrill from mitral stenosis. Increased amplitude (pounding) at the apex may be from a thin, flat, or depressed sternum.

A heart with an apex displaced to the left is almost sure to be enlarged. When the pulsation is very strong, you may be able to auscultate a gallop rhythm. Report it to the doctor.

Pulsations in the *epigastric area* are common in anemic or feverish children. Pulsations can also mean tricuspid stenosis, tricuspid regurgitation, or thyrotoxicosis.

Pulmonary

Aortic

Right ventricular

Apical
Epigastric

Listen for murmurs
Evaluate all murmurs carefully and record them as to their timing, location, radiation, intensity, pitch, and quality. Murmurs can be innocent (or functional) or organic. They can be so soft as to be almost inaudible (Grade I) or may be loud enough to be heard with the stethoscope off the chest wall (Grade VI). But only the most experienced listeners can decide whether they are innocent or not. Yet there are some clues you can keep in mind. Innocent murmurs are usually systolic, soft (Grade I or II), and transient. They are usually located at the pulmonic area, and are not transmitted. All have in common: absence of symptoms or any sign of heart disease on physical exam, EKG, or chest X-ray. They do not affect growth and development. But even these clues are not foolproof. Children with murmurs always need careful cardiac evaluation.

tributed crunching noise resulting from air in the mediastinum. It is rare but always needs attention. Report it promptly.

Clicks, splits, and hums

You may also hear clicks and ejection noises. A pulmonary ejection click is localized at the base, the anterior precordium; it lessens during inspiration or becomes louder during expiration. Pulmonary hypertension, ventricular septal defect, patent ductus, atrial septal defect, or pulmonary stenosis can cause it. An aortic ejection click occurs in early systole at the base and at the apex: This does not change with respiration. It can be caused by aortic coarctation, aneurysm, or valve stenosis. An opening snap resembles a click, but has a different quality. This sound occurs, when it does, soon after S_2 in the third or fourth left intercostal space. It results from mitral stenosis or an atrial tumor (such as myxoma).

Or you might hear one of two kinds of splits. The first is a split of the first heart sound. Remember the first heart sound reflects closure of tricuspid and mitral valves. The mitral valve closes a small fraction of a second ahead of the tricuspid, but in most people, the timing is so close that they sound like one. In some people, this sounds like a distinctly double beat over the left sternal border. It's probably normal. But if you hear a wide split, or hear it in other areas — particularly at the apex — report it.

You may hear a venous hum, a continuous, low-pitched hum heard throughout the cycle, but loudest during diastole. You can hear it best at the supraclavicular fossae, but you can also pick it up in the second to third intercostal space on both sides of the sternum. Not usually affected by respiration, this hum may sound louder when the child is standing. You can obliterate it by turning the child's head, or occluding his carotid pulse with your fingers. This hum is almost always normal, but may mèan thyrotoxicosis or anemia.

Cardiac Babies
Know six common anomalies

BY KATHY MURPHY, RN, BSN, MSN and
KIT STAHLER, RN, BSN, MSN

WHEN A FULL-TERM BABY with a malformed heart survives his first month of life, he is one of only about two hundred such survivors his age in this country. For every such living baby, another one will have died. But at least half of those who died might at least have been candidates for corrective surgery — if their heart defects had been detected early enough.

Some heart defects do not show up for several years. But roughly 1% of newborns have heart defects severe enough to produce symptoms. If you work in pediatrics, or even plan to, you should know what these symptoms are and what they mean. Do you know why symptoms of congenital heart disease appear in a seemingly healthy toddler or newborn? How to assess such children accurately? Before you can answer these questions, you must understand the effects of oxygen saturation and pressure on cardiac lesions.

Oxygen saturation is simply a relative measurement (expressed as a percentage) of the amount of oxygen the hemoglobin can carry. In the normal heart, venous (right-sided) oxygen saturation is low because the tissues have extracted oxygen from this blood to meet metabolic demands; on the left side, the freshly oxygenated arterial saturation is higher because it carries deliverable oxygen to the tissues.

Pressure involves flow and resistance. Each of the four chambers in the heart has a different blood pressure (see below). Because the atria are essentially collection chambers, pressures in the atria are lower there than in the more muscular ventricles. Pressures in the left side of the heart are higher because the left ventricle pumps against high systemic resistance. The right ventricle pumps against lower pulmonary resistance and, therefore, has a lower pressure than the left ventricle. It's important to remember this. When an abnormal

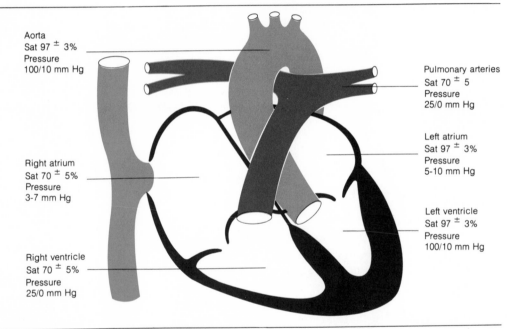

Aorta
Sat 97 ± 3%
Pressure
100/10 mm Hg

Pulmonary arteries
Sat 70 ± 5
Pressure
25/0 mm Hg

Left atrium
Sat 97 ± 3%
Pressure
5-10 mm Hg

Right atrium
Sat 70 ± 5%
Pressure
3-7 mm Hg

Left ventricle
Sat 97 ± 3%
Pressure
100/10 mm Hg

Right ventricle
Sat 70 ± 5%
Pressure
25/0 mm Hg

What's normal?
Pressures and oxygen saturation values in the heart of a newborn, as shown here, differ from those of an adult, shown on page 52.

communication exists in the heart, blood *always* flows (or shunts) from an area of higher to lower pressure.

Knowing these differences in oxygen saturation and pressure, and the structural anomalies in congenital defects, you can predict the changes in blood flow each defect can produce. With this in mind, you can plan appropriate nursing care for children with congenital heart disease. Let's review these factors in the six most common congenital defects.

Four acyanotic defects
1. *Ventricular septal defect (VSD),* the most common congen-

Fetal shunts
In the circulation of a fetus, special shunts — the foramen ovale, the ductus arteriosus, and the ductus venosus — allow most of the blood to bypass the immature liver and lungs which do not yet function fully.

Ductus arteriosus

Foramen ovale

Ductus venosus

SIX MOST COMMON ANOMALIES

VENTRICULAR SEPTAL DEFECT (VSD)
One or more openings between the ventricles.

CIRCULATORY CONSIDERATIONS
Acyanotic defect: Blood flows from area of higher to area of lower concentration. This left to right shunt may cause pulmonary congestion and pulmonary artery hypertension.

MURMUR
Heard in lower left sternal border, may be associated with palpable thrill. Auscultory findings depend on size of defect and the amount of pulmonary vascular resistance.

TREATMENT
Medical: CHF regimen (sedation, rest, oxygen, digoxin, sodium restriction, diuretics).
Surgical: Simple closure or patch on cardiopulmonary bypass (corrective).

ATRIAL SEPTAL DEFECT (ASD)
One or more openings between the atria. Includes ostium secundum, ostium primum, and sinus venosus.

CIRCULATORY CONSIDERATIONS
Acyanotic defect. Left to right shunt may cause pulmonary congestion and pulmonary artery hypertension. Atrial arrhythmias secondary to right atrial overload and resultant interference with conduction system.

MURMUR
Systolic ejection is greatest in second and third left intercostal spaces.
Fixed split S_2 on expiration heard in second, third, or fourth intercostal space.

TREATMENT
Medical: Not usually necessary.
Surgical: Direct closure or patch graft on cardiopulmonary bypass.

PATENT DUCTUS ARTERIOSUS (PDA)
Opening between the descending aorta and bifurcation of the pulmonary artery.

CIRCULATORY CONSIDERATIONS
Acyanotic defect. Left to right shunt may cause pulmonary congestion and pulmonary artery hypertension. Increased incidence in premature infants. Pulse pressure may be widened; pulses full or bounding.

MURMUR
Continuous "machinery" murmur, greatest at upper left sternal border and under clavicle.

TREATMENT
Medical: CHF regimen, Indomethacin, Rashkind plugging procedure.
Surgical: Ductal ligation, in severe cases when infant is 3 to 4 days old; otherwise during toddler age to prevent pulmonary hypertension.

SIX MOST COMMON ANOMALIES

COARCTATION OF THE AORTA
Constriction of descending aorta near the ductus arteriosus.

CIRCULATORY CONSIDERATIONS
Acyanotic defect. Elevated pressures in ascending aorta and left ventricle. Insufficient mitral valve. Back pressure to lungs. Aneurysms, increased blood pressure in upper extremities, and leg cramping (may be confused with growing pains).

MURMUR
Systolic ejection click heard at base and apex of heart. Associated with systolic or continuous murmur between scapulae.

TREATMENT
Medical: CHF regimen, exercise restriction.
Surgical: Resection and anastomosis, performed when patient is 7 to 10 years old.

TETRALOGY OF FALLOT
Four defects: VSD, overriding aorta, pulmonary stenosis, and right ventricular hypertrophy.

CIRCULATORY CONSIDERATIONS
Pulmonary stenosis restricts blood flow to lungs. Unoxygenated blood is shunted through the VSD. Saturated and unsaturated blood is mixed in the left ventricle and is pumped out the aorta, producing cyanosis, Tet spells, clubbing, squatting.

MURMUR
Single S2 systolic murmur greatest in second and third intercostal spaces at left sternal border.

TREATMENT
Medical: CHF regimen
Surgical: Palliative — Pott's, Blalock-Taussig, Waterston. Corrective — Close VSD and relieve pulmonary stenosis.

TRANSPOSITION OF GREAT VESSELS
Aorta leaves right ventricle, pulmonary artery leaves left ventricle.

CIRCULATORY CONSIDERATIONS
Unoxygenated blood flows through right atrium and ventricle and out aorta to systemic circulation again. Oxygenated blood flows from lungs to left atrium and ventricle and out pulmonary artery to lungs. Sudden severe cyanosis.

MURMUR
Loud aortic closure sound at second left intercostal space. Systolic murmur heard if VSD is present.

TREATMENT
Medical: Balloon septostomy, CHF regimen.
Surgical: Palliative — Blalock-Hanlon. Corrective — Mustard procedure.

Cyanosis

The blue tint of cyanosis under the skin and mucous membranes comes from an abnormally high level of deoxygenated hemoglobin in capillary beds. The neonate's normal levels of hemoglobin are 16 to 22 grams/100 ml although after 1 year they will have dropped to 12 grams/100 ml. Normally 95 to 98% of this hemoglobin oxidizes in the lungs to oxyhemoglobin. With valvular or lung obstruction, extra openings in the heart chambers, or a weak pump, oxidation may be less complete. When deoxygenated levels reach 3 to 4 gram/100 ml, you may see mild cyanosis. When they climb to about 5 gram/100 ml, you'll see frank cyanosis.

Peripheral cyanosis characterizes low cardiac output. With sluggish circulation, the peripheral capillary bed constricts. In compensation, tissues extract more oxygen from the blood, leaving more deoxygenated hemoglobin.

Central cyanosis comes from inadequate oxygenation. Congenital heart defects can cause it. Pulmonary disease or obstruction leads to inadequate oxygenation at the alveolar-capillary site; this delivers less than fully saturated blood to the left atrium. The venous blood, shunted from right to left through a septal defect or a patent ductus that bypasses the lungs, may dilute the oxygen levels of the blood in the systemic circuit. In other words, abnormally deoxygenated blood is delivered to tissues which extract so much more oxygen that cyanosis becomes evident.

ital defect, allows oxygenated blood to shunt from the left to the right ventricle. Such defects may be large enough to obliterate the septum and require surgical repair. But many are small enough to close spontaneously. The opening's size and its effect on the pulmonary vasculature (the degree of congestion) determine severity of symptoms and resultant management. Tony's case was typical.

Tony is a 10-month-old infant in the cardiac clinic for progressive congestive heart failure (CHF) associated with a moderate VSD. Tony seems small but is appropriately active for his age. His mother says he's gained weight very slowly despite a good appetite. She says she fed him solid foods at 2 months because he had trouble bottle-feeding. During feedings, he needed several rest periods, became dyspneic, and sweated profusely.

While Tony sits quietly on his mother's lap, he shows no acute distress. But when he cries, he becomes dyspneic and shows mild intercostal retractions and flaring nares. Tony doesn't become cyanotic when he cries, but he does become very pale. If you listened to his apical heart rate, you'd find that it increased dramatically with activity, from 100 at rest to more than 160 when crying. You'd hear a coarse systolic heart murmur at his lower left sternal border and bilateral fine moist rales at the end of the inspiration. Depending on the size of the defect, you might palpate a thrill and a prominent precordial bulge. Although Tony's liver is palpable 2.5 cm below his right costal margin, he does not have edema.

Tony shows many signs common to children with right-sided congestive heart failure (see p. 26). Indeed, most children like Tony receive treatment only after developing signs of congestive heart failure. Surgical correction is usually postponed, if possible, for two reasons: Some VSDs close spontaneously and, even if they do not, children tolerate heart surgery better after the age of 4.

Total correction of septal defects is done with simple closure (small to moderate defects) or by placement of a patch graft (large defects).

2. *Atrial septal defect (ASD),* the second most common anomaly, is an abnormal opening between the atria. It causes changes in blood flow similar to those in VSD except for the volume of blood shunted. Because of lower pressure in the atria, ASD shunts less blood from the left to the right side.

Consequently, ASD rarely causes congestive heart failure in young children. However, the decreased systemic cardiac output from the ASD fails to deliver optimal oxygen and nutrients to the tissues. This results in impaired growth so children with ASD tend to be small for their age. Also, pulmonary overload (interstitial edema), predisposes the child to frequent respiratory infections.

Left-to-right shunts initially markedly increase pulmonary blood flow. Overcirculation of this vasculature may gradually make the vessels fibrotic and less elastic. This change produces hypertension within the pulmonary circuit and eventually reverses the intracardiac shunt from right to left.

ASD is usually corrected in late childhood to prevent permanent pulmonary vascular changes associated with pulmonary overload.

3. *Patent ductus arteriosus (PDA),* a remnant of fetal circulation (see p. 26), is an opening between the aorta and pulmonary artery. Its fetal purpose is to shunt blood away from the nonfunctional (collapsed) lungs. The ductus arteriosus normally closes spontaneously soon after birth (usually within 72 hours, but may take as long as 2 weeks). Failure to close (PDA) occurs most often in premature infants. Such infants may develop congestive heart failure because the left-to-right shunt increases blood flow to the lungs and left atrium.

Sam is a 4-month-old infant admitted for surgical ligation of a PDA. His medical records show that he was 6 weeks premature and that he required vigorous treatment (including mechanical ventilation) for respiratory distress syndrome — a disease secondary to lung immaturity.

Sam's congestive heart failure was managed with oral digitalis b.i.d. His mother says the doctors hoped digitalis would support his cardiac function until spontaneous closure of the PDA could occur. But this was a vain hope. Sam developed severe symptoms of right heart failure, similar to Tony's. If you could examine Sam, you'd see that he became dyspneic with the least exertion. You'd see tachypnea, intercostal retractions, and flaring nares; and palpate bounding axillary, femoral, and pedal pulses, and feel a thrill over his chest wall — all suggesting an A-V fistula (a runoff from the aorta to the pulmonary artery).

Sam will have surgical ligation of his PDA as soon as medical management brings his CHF under control. PDA is gener-

Fingers and toes
These photographs show the clubbing of the digits commonly associated with congenital heart disease, in this case with tetralogy of Fallot.

The stricken heart

A failing heart can no longer pump enough blood to meet the body's metabolic needs. When the left ventricle can't eject the volume presented to it, blood dams up behind it, engorging the pulmonary vasculature. The lungs lose compliance and adequate gas exchange requires more effort. Recognize left heart failure by its classic signs: labored breathing with flaring nostrils, restlessness, and apprehension. Yet, in infants, tachypnea may be the only sign of impending heart failure. A sustained increase of 10 breaths a minute in a quiet, sleeping baby becomes significant. So watch for changes in respiratory rate.

In right heart failure, systemic engorgement produces distended neck veins, hepatosplenomegaly, edema of the legs (in an older child or an adult), and presacral edema. But in an infant, edema of the eyelids or face may be the first sign of heart failure (or of excessive fluid administration). Generally recumbent, infants are less likely to develop leg edema. Watch for swollen eyelids and features.

Treat heart failure with:
• sedation (usually morphine) to reduce anxiety and irritability
• rest to lighten the heart's work
• oxygen to saturate the blood and maintain tissue perfusion
• digitalis to increase the heart's power of contraction
• sodium restriction to reduce fluid retention
• diuretics to lessen edema.

ally corrected earlier than VSD because such ligation is a closed-heart procedure which doesn't require cardiopulmonary bypass and involves less risk.

4. *Coarctation of the aorta* most commonly occurs as a narrowing of the descending aorta in the area of the ductus arteriosus. It causes elevated pressures in the ascending aorta and left ventricle which create mitral regurgitation and back pressure to the lungs. CHF may result. The increased pressure in the ascending aorta produces elevated blood pressures in the arms with possible headaches, nosebleeds, flushed cheeks, CVAs (from aneurysms, thrombosis, emboli) and lower blood pressure in the legs.

Steve, 9 years old, illustrates symptoms unique to coarctation of the aorta. Steve's school nurse first suspected his coarctation during a preschool physical examination. She noticed mild hypertension (140/100) in his arms associated with hypotension (70/50) in his legs. She palpated his pulses and found bilateral equal and full brachial pulses, weak femorals, and bilateral absence of his pedal pulses. She referred him for cardiac evaluation which confirmed coarctation. Since then, Steve has been healthy and has developed normally. However, because of the risk of myocardial ischemia associated with vigorous exercise, Steve has been restricted from competitive sports.

To identify children like Steve, practice good techniques for taking blood pressure in children. Always assure proper cuff size for arms and legs. Record blood pressures from all four extremities and compare the quality of brachial, radial, femoral, popliteal, and pedal pulses bilaterally. Observe for flushed cheeks and remember to ask children about headaches or nosebleeds.

Surgical repair of coarctation is usually postponed until the child is 6 to 12 years old, because the anastomosis site does not grow proportionately with length of the aorta. Thus, postponement prevents a second surgical repair.

Two cyanotic defects

5. *Tetralogy of Fallot* includes four structural anomalies: ventricular septal defect (VSD); dextroposition or overriding of the aorta; right ventricular outflow obstruction or pulmonary stenosis; and right ventricular hypertrophy. Of the four defects, pulmonary stenosis and VSD are the most important

because they cause cyanosis. The pulmonary stenosis causes right ventricular hypertrophy. This causes unoxygenated blood to be shunted through the VSD into the left ventricle where it is mixed. Thus, the ventricle pumps arterial blood with an abnormally low oxygen saturation to the systemic tissues and causes cyanosis.

Let's look at Amy, 2 years old, with confirmed tetralogy of Fallot. Her cardiac defects were confirmed by cardiac catheterization at age 3 months. Her medical management has been successful so far. But now, Amy's mother becomes very apprehensive whenever Amy shows any signs of distress. She's afraid Amy will have another "blue spell" ("tet spell") and that she might die. She says these spells are usually unpredictable, but that some happen after breakfast. During these spells, Amy becomes dyspneic and restless, her cyanosis deepens, and she gasps for breath. Usually, these spells can be relieved by placing Amy in a knee-chest position.

Recently Amy had a "blue spell" that left her unconscious but breathing for about 3 minutes. She was rushed to the emergency department where she was found to be alert, reactive, mildly dyspneic, and cyanotic. Blood studies at that time showed mild acidosis (pH 7.30) and polycythemia (hematocrit 65%). Amy was admitted for cardiac evaluation. If she'd had a severe "tet spell" while hospitalized, treatment would have included 100% oxygen by anesthesia mask to relieve hypoxia; morphine subcutaneously, to calm her and break the dyspnea cycle; sodium bicarbonate to correct acidosis; and, possibly, propranolol (Inderal) to relieve acute dyspneic attacks.

If you could observe Amy, you'd see obvious cyanosis even when she's resting. The cyanosis looks deepest in her lips and nailbeds, but all of her skin has a dusky, bluish cast. She's slightly dyspneic. Her fingernails and toenails are clubbed, and she's small for her age.

She's small because she uses up so much of her energy (oxygen and calories) just for normal activities such as feeding and for coping with dyspnea, increased cardiac activity, and recurrent infection. Her dyspnea and cyanosis increase with feeding, defecation, and stress. Her "blue spells" are most likely when she's crying or has an infection.

Children like Amy know their own exercise limitations. Typically, they play and walk for a while but soon stop and squat while resting. Squatting decreases venous return and

Clues to congenital heart abnormalities

IN INFANTS
dyspnea
difficulty with feeding
   (falls asleep after taking only 2 oz. of formula)
stridor or choking spell
pulse rate over 160
recurrent respiratory infections
failure to gain weight
heart murmurs
cyanosis
anoxic attacks

IN CHILDREN
dyspnea
poor physical development
decreased exercise tolerance
recurrent respiratory infections
heart murmur and thrill
cyanosis
squatting
clubbing of fingers and toes
elevated blood pressure

The goals of home care

Many parents need support to accept their child's defect immediately after his birth. Help them express their feelings so they can cope more effectively. Reassure them about caring for a special child. Tell them what problems to expect and how to meet them:

• Such a child will be smaller than normal — not because of incorrect nurturing, assure them, but because incomplete oxygenation hinders growth.

• Such infants need more time for feedings and need to start solid foods earlier, which takes less energy than sucking a bottle. Suggest small frequent feedings rich in iron.

• Warn parents against overprotection. Such children naturally know their own limits.

• Explain the medications their child needs, the purposes, doses, and side effects. Most children with CHD need digoxin to strengthen the heart's contractions. Remind parents to give only the *exact amount prescribed at the right time by mouth* and not to mix it with foods. Have them watch for signs of digitalis toxicity. Also, remind them to replace the potassium wasted by diuretics.

• Low-sodium diets may make the child a problem eater. Suggest appealing substitutes.

• Children with cardiac defects, vulnerable to respiratory infections, must avoid people with colds.

• Congestive heart failure usually develops slowly, over days. But review the danger signs: sustained increased respirations, excessive sweating, irritability and distress associated with exercise.

increases systemic resistance to lessen the right-to-left shunt, to improve oxygen saturation.

Amy has frequent respiratory infections because the right-to-left shunt allows much of her circulating blood to bypass the lungs' cleansing filtration. She has persistent polycythemia because her bone marrow compensates for low arterial oxygen saturation by producing more oxygen carriers — RBCs.

The increasing severity and frequency of Amy's "blue spells," coupled with polycythemia, make her a candidate for corrective surgery. Because her cyanosis results partially from a mechanical inability to perfuse her lungs, a palliative shunt may be created to increase blood flow to her lungs. Such palliative procedures (Blalock-Taussig, Waterston, and Pott's) are closed-heart methods. Total correction (with closure of VSD and relief of pulmonary stenosis) requires cardiopulmonary bypass and may be postponed until a better time.

6. *Transposition of the great vessels* occurs when the great arteries are reversed: The aorta arises from the right ventricle and the pulmonary artery arises from the left ventricle. This produces two noncommunicating circulatory systems — a condition incompatible with life. A child with this defect needs a shunt to bridge the arterial and venous systems and mix high-oxygen saturated blood from the left heart with low-oxygen saturated blood in the right heart. In the first few days of life, such an infant benefits from the patent ductus arteriosus. However, in a few days when this temporary pathway closes spontaneously, he quickly deteriorates. His survival depends on rapid identification of his defect and appropriate treatment.

Diane, 7 days old, was admitted 2 nights ago with a diagnosis of transposition. She was vigorous at birth with a 5-minute Apgar score of 7 to 9. She was pink and had no symptoms until the third day. Then, nurses noticed that she needed extra time for feeding and became pale, tachypneic, and tachycardic when crying. Over the next 2 days, these symptoms became worse and she became dusky with stress. On the fifth day, she suddenly became deeply cyanotic and distressed. An emergency balloon septostomy created an ASD which relieved her distress. It will allow adequate oxygenation until she can have corrective surgery.

3

Cardiac Surgery
Know how to cope

BY KIT STAHLER, RN, BSN, MSN and
KATHY MURPHY, RN, BSN, MSN

DAVID, 6 YEARS OLD, is admitted for surgical closure of a large ventricular septal defect (VSD). He's one of a growing number of children hospitalized for surgical correction of congenital heart defects.

Would you feel competent to care for a child like David? To prepare him psychologically and physically for surgery? And keep track of his condition after surgery? To helpfully involve his parents? Here are some ways to do all those things well.

Your goals vary
Before surgery, your goals include preparing the child for surgery — first psychologically by telling him what to expect before, during, and after surgery — without intensifying his anxiety. Then you physically prepare him, while offering emotional support and reassurance. And you must prepare his parents to support and reassure him throughout this terrifying crisis.

After surgery, you must know how to monitor his condition for physiological stability; what complications to watch for and how to recognize them; what drugs will be given and how to use them safely. And, of course, you must prepare parents to care for him during his convalescence at home. Let's look at these goals in more detail.

Expect problems at admission

Children like David are usually admitted 2 to 5 days before surgery to prepare them emotionally and physically, and to complete routine studies. Many hospitals give them and their parents a tour of the unit and information about the surgery. Even after such orientation, you'll find most children and their parents in a highly anxious state.

Parents like David's have known for a long time that surgery was inevitable for his survival. They've surely tried to prepare themselves and their child for this frightening event. Still, they can't help feeling overwhelmed by their fear of what may happen.

Parents with any unresolved guilt or inability to accept the child's defect will have much difficulty. They'll show it by being very demanding — asking many questions... looking for frequent attention for seemingly insignificant things and reasons...and even acting hostile. You need to realize this is not directed at you personally. Try to spend time with them. Allow them to express their anxiety, guilt, and frustrations. Doing so will help the child indirectly; his anxiety will, to some extent, mirror theirs.

Also remember the many sources of the child's anxiety. Many children David's age view hospitalization and painful procedures as punishment for misbehavior or bad thoughts. They are still egocentric. David's anxiety may be rooted in fear of: separation from his parents, loss of parental love, punishment, or physical harm. He may fear needles, cuts, and foreign objects on his body. He may have a heightened awareness of his body, an exaggerated concern for privacy, and may be overly modest — refuse hospital gowns, "forget" to save urine specimens, shun rectal temperatures, and deny constipation.

Older school-age children may fear abandonment, body mutilation, and death. But don't go by chronological age alone. It may be misleading. Regression is a normal and expected defense mechanism at any age: It allows the threatened person to fall back on earlier coping mechanisms. But it is frightening. The child who regresses realizes his immature inclinations, but cannot accept or control his response.

Plan teaching sessions

Before you actually begin teaching a child like David, carefully assess his and his parents' understanding of the situation and the ability of them all to cope. Look for their strengths and weaknesses. Then, explain everything to child and parents together. This helps the child feel more secure and helps the parents reinforce the information.

Gear your teaching to the child's developmental level and his ability to absorb any new information. If he is too anxious, he won't learn. For example, if he looks away, walks around the room, or begins to play while you're talking to him — he's had enough. When you *do* have his attention, build on what he already knows. Proceed from simple to complex explanations and talk about nonthreatening activities first. Save descriptions of threatening events (like needles) until just before they occur. Make teaching sessions short; use dolls, miniature equipment, and photographs.

Take David and his parents on a tour of the operating room (mainly by photographs) and ICU. Introduce him to his ICU nurse. If possible, also introduce him to another child close to his age who's had similar surgery. This may help reassure him that he will be alright. Emphasize that not every piece of equipment that he sees will be used on him — just the ones you tell him about.

Give simple, honest reasons for treatments and activities. Never lie. If you lie to manipulate a child into cooperation, you'll destroy his trust and create serious problems. Honest explanations before painful procedures usually increase a child's tolerance of them. Be sensitive to unasked questions. Also remember, the little things can upset children the most, like needles...not being able to have orange juice the morning of surgery...and not being able to wear underpants in the ICU.

Don't forget to tell parents how long surgery will probably last. Explain that the first 2 hours of surgery involve anesthesia, cooling, and placement of tubes. The actual corrective procedure may take less than an hour. Then, closure and rewarming will take an additional 2 hours. During surgery, try to provide brief progress reports to ease the stress of waiting.

Preoperative preparation

Physical preoperative preparation may include:
- cardiac catheterization to evaluate cardiac status

Things to tell children before cardiac surgery
- What sights and sounds (alarms and so forth) to expect in the operating room and intensive care unit.
- Monitoring equipment won't hurt.
- Catheters and monitoring equipment will be placed while he's under anesthesia and will be removed as he gets better.
- Blood on dressings and in chest tubes after surgery is normal and to be expected.
- Endotracheal intubation (call it a breathing tube) will allow periodic suctioning and it will cause him to lose his voice temporarily. Assure him that nurses will be near at all times and can read lips.
- A tube will drain urine into a bag (so he shouldn't worry about wetting the bed).
- Restraint is for protection, not punishment. Without restraint, he might pull out some of his equipment during his sleep.
- He'll be sore when he wakes up after surgery. He should tell his nurse whenever he hurts so she can give him pain medication.
- Parents will visit often, but sometimes he'll have to wait to see them.

• blood studies (CBC, BUN, and creatinine to assess renal function)
• electrolytes
• arterial blood gases (ABGs)
• coagulation profile, and type and crossmatch for donor blood
• urinalysis to evaluate his renal function
• getting an accurate weight (used to calculate fluids, electrolytes, volume replacement, and medication doses). Congestive heart failure and infections must be controlled before surgery. Some children may be given prophylactic antibiotics.

The immediate preoperative preparation varies. Some hospitals require routine antibacterial skin-cleanser baths or showers several days in advance. Others require a Betadine wash or scrub on the day before surgery. The skin shave is done from neck to knees. Tell David about the skin prep and the cleansing enema just before doing them. Afterward, explain why he can't eat or drink for a while afterwards, why wearing a hospital gown is necessary, how he'll be transported (bed or stretcher), and who'll go to the operating room with him. Explain that the preop medication will make him sleepy. Don't say it will "*put* him to sleep"; some children associate that with death.

Postoperative monitoring vital

Immediately after surgery, nursing care includes close observation and frequent reassessment of the child's physical condition. As soon as a child like David arrives from surgery, assess his cardiovascular status. His heart rate should be 70 to 100 and regular. (Heart rates for other children should be within normal limits for their age.) Monitor for arrhythmias and get a rhythm strip hourly. Arrhythmias can be expected because of surgical trauma to the conduction system, prolonged cardiopulmonary bypass, digoxin therapy, or potassium imbalance. Like some children, David could need temporary transvenous pacing.

Palpate and compare all his peripheral pulses to assess cardiac function. Dangerous signs of poor cardiac output: cool, clammy skin; mottling; poor capillary refill; and urine output less than 1 ml/kg/hour.

After cardiac surgery, David had intracardiac catheters, (CVP, PAP/wedge) connected to an oscilloscope to measure

Aftermath of cardiac surgery

Recovering from cardiac surgery is an enormous job. A child can easily become overwhelmed by the strange environment and frightening equipment. Here are some things you can do to make his course easier.

First, cope with your own anxiety so you don't pass it along to your patient. Know what to expect so you're prepared for any situation.

Second, to make the child feel more comfortable and less lost, place toys and other familiar objects from home within his sight.

Third, talk to your patient when you give physical care. Reassure him with a touch or by the tone of your voice that everything will be OK.

Fourth, hospitalized children can be comforted by hearing the voices of family and friends on a cassette tape recorder.

Show that you care

Even the best prepared child will feel lost and frightened in a hospital situation. You can foster some sense of security by continually reassuring him by words and actions that you will try to meet his needs.

For example, assure his comfort by controlling pain. Give pain medication half an hour before painful procedures and whenever he seems restless or cannot sleep. Relieving pain helps prevent feelings of anger and loss of control and encourages cooperation.

Remember that immobility, multiple tubes, and the imposition of treatments can cause feelings of helplessness. So return as much control as possible. Offer simple choices like asking your patient when he wants to bathe or sit in a chair. This allows him to cope in his own way with unpleasant situations.

Above all, involve parents in nursing care whenever possible. This helps fill parental needs and fosters security for them and the child.

blood pressures within his various heart chambers. Report all variations from normal limits. Watch for an increased CVP (central venous pressure) associated with decreased intra-arterial pressure, or increased pulmonary artery pressure and other signs of left-sided heart failure (frothy endotracheal secretions, dyspnea, cough, and pulmonary rales). Heart failure may be secondary to volume overload and a damaged conduction system.

Another postop problem to worry about: cardiac tamponade. It occurs when the heart gets compressed in the mediastinal space by clotted or unclotted blood and can't function effectively as a pump. *It's an extreme emergency* and requires immediate thoracentesis or thoracotomy. Watch for its signs: sudden increase or decrease in the chest tube drainage accompanied by decreased blood pressure, narrowed pulse pressure, increased CVP, engorged neck veins, and pulsus paradoxus (a marked decrease in pulse amplitude with inspiration).

If David was receiving digoxin, the doctor may order it resumed postoperatively. *Caution:* Because of the hazards of digoxin in persons with hypokalemia, always get *a serum potassium before beginning digoxin treatment*. Thereafter, check the serum potassium level every 2 to 3 days, or as ordered.

Respiratory care vital

Note whether David's respirations are spontaneous or respirator-dependent. They should be regular at a rate of 20 to 22 per minute. Watch for signs of respiratory distress — tachypnea, dyspnea, retractions, flaring nares, grunting, prolonged expiration, duskiness, or cyanosis. Look for bilateral equal expansion of his chest wall. Auscultate breath sounds for bilateral equality of aeration, absence of aeration in any area(s), or accessory sounds such as rales, rhonchi, or rubs (over the anterior chest). Monitor arterial blood gases to assess ability to oxygenate and remove CO_2.

Pneumothorax is a potential complication of both cardiac surgery and mechanical ventilation. A tension pneumothorax is a collection of air under pressure in the pleural space which compromises lung expansion. Suspect it when you find an absence of breath sounds accompanied by a gradual or sudden increase in dyspnea. Prompt insertion of a chest tube can reestablish the negative intrapleural pressure and help to relieve distress.

At most hospitals, a portable chest X-ray is used immediately after surgery and then daily to view lung reexpansion and heart size. Two chest tubes (one, a mediastinal tube) are generally in place. These tubes are usually connected to a portable drainage system which is connected to wall suction. These tubes need frequent and careful milking or stripping to prevent clot formation. Record the amount, color, and consistency of the drainage hourly. Total these amounts at the end of your shift and record them in your notes. Tape the same information on the Pleur-evac with your initials, the time, and the date.

Watch for complications
Guard against hypovolemia, a frequent complication due to inadequate postoperative blood replacement. To evaluate the adequacy of blood and fluid replacement, monitor intracardiac pressures, the amounts of chest tube drainage, and urine output. Hypovolemia can lead to poor renal perfusion and renal shutdown. So, maintain adequate urine output. Body weight is the final index of fluid balance, so weigh the child daily at the same time each day, on a bedside scale.

Check serum electrolytes. Initially, you'll need to check David's electrolytes at least every 4 hours because rapid shifts can occur. You may see hyponatremia (dilutional) which the doctor will treat with diuretics and decreased water intake. However, you must watch most zealously for electrolyte shifts that may cause arrhythmias. Hyperkalemia may cause premature ventricular contractions (PVCs) and cardiac arrest. And, hypokalemia and hypocalcemia intensify the patient's sensitivity to digoxin (Lanoxin).

Monitor hematologic studies. Hemoglobin and hematocrit are indexes of hydration as well as other functions. Clotting studies (prothrombin time and partial thromboplastin time) are ordered to check reversal of heparinization by protamine during surgery. The platelet count tells the degree of platelet destruction by the membrane oxygenator. The BUN (blood urea nitrogen) and creatinine provide an index of renal function.

Assess neurological status. Complications of the membrane oxygenator are thrombi, emboli, and cerebral anoxic damage. All can impair neurologic function. Repeatedly evaluate pupil equality and reaction to light, equal movement and sensation in extremities, level of consciousness, and response to commands.

Convalescence after ICU

A patient like David will probably need treatment in the ICU for at least 2 days. As he improves, his supportive equipment will be removed. Then, he and his parents may need reassurance that intensive monitoring and observation are no longer necessary and that he can be cared for just as well on the regular floor.

Children like David need postoperative care for about another week before they can be discharged. Nursing care during this early convalescence includes observation for, and prevention of, infection in the incisional areas; chest hygiene (postural drainage and percussion to maintain pulmonary functions and prevent respiratory infections); continued assessment of breath sounds (the doctor will investigate decreased aeration in any area by X-ray to rule out pneumonia); and regular cardiovascular assessments.

Maintaining fluid and electrolyte balance remains important during early convalescence. The child may need fluid restriction and a low-sodium diet to decrease the workload on the healing heart muscle; he may be discharged on this special diet. Be sure to explain the reason for this and other restrictions to the parents during your discharge teaching.

Prepare the parents for his convalescence at home. Tell them what temporary behavior problems he may show at home. While recovering from the severe trauma of surgery, he may regress, whine, cling, or be emotionally labile; he may lose his appetite and have nightmares. When the family expects and understands this, they can be more patient and accepting. Of course, if such problems continue for longer than a few months, parents should consult their pediatrician.

Remember to send a progress report to the child's school nurse to ease the transition back to school.

SKILLCHECK 1

1. Sally, 6 months old, is admitted to your pediatric unit for cardiac evaluation. Her skin looks dusky when she cries. When you take her pulse, you feel a forceful bounding quality over both the radial and femoral pulses. What diagnosis do you suspect?

2. When you take Sally's blood pressure, you hear pulse sounds begin, become muffled, and then disappear. Which point is the diastolic blood pressure?

3. Bill, 9 months old, is hospitalized for upper respiratory infection. When you listen to his heart, you notice that S_1 and S_2 are followed by a distinct low-pitched sound that you hear best at the apex. What is it and what should you do about it?

4. Tommy is 9 years old. When you take his apical pulse, you notice that his heart rate speeds up with inspiration and slows down with expiration. What does this mean?

5. Which of the following is *not* a symptom of cardiac disease in a 3-month-old infant: falling asleep after taking 2 oz. of milk; clubbing of fingers and toes; S_3 on auscultation; or failure to gain weight?

6. In children, a narrow pulse pressure (less than 20 mm Hg) suggests which of the following: patent ductus arteriosus; aortic stenosis; tetralogy of Fallot; or aortic regurgitation?

7. In children born with tetralogy of Fallot, a common compensation by the body for low arterial oxygen saturation is... fatigue, high blood pressure, right ventricular hypertrophy, or polycythemia?

8. Children with cardiac defects are often hospitalized with respiratory infections. Why are they susceptible to these infections? Is the mechanism the same in acyanotic and cyanotic disorders?

9. Following cardiac surgery, cool and clammy skin, poor capillary refill, and low urine output are ominous signs of: decreased renal function, cardiac tamponade, hypertensive crisis, or low cardiac output?

10. Paul has just returned from surgery where his ventricular septal defect was repaired. You notice that he is having 6 to 10 PVCs (premature ventricular contractions) per minute. What does this mean and what should you do?

(Answers on page 171)

IN ADULTS:

DEAL WITH ACQUIRED DISEASE

4

Assessment
Review of vital skills

BY CHRISTINE SUE BREU, RN, BSN, MN

CAREFUL ASSESSMENT IS ONE of your most vital contributions
to the care of patients with cardiovascular problems. During
the initial assessment, it's your assignment to collect all pertinent information about the patient's present condition and his
medical history. This careful evaluation helps pinpoint the
source of the problems; sets a reliable baseline against which
to measure the effectiveness of treatment; and helps you to
plan comprehensive care.

Don't overlook the history
In haste to identify the patient's problems, you may be tempted to overlook the medical history. Yet, the subjective information the patient himself can give you may be crucial. Always remember to define the patient's chief complaint — the
patient's description in his own words of what caused him to
seek medical help. You might ask "What brought you to the
hospital (or doctor's office)?" or, "What is your problem?"
Then find out how long he's had this problem, the details
surrounding its onset, and any causative factors. Be sure to
elicit a full description of the symptoms, the locations, radiation, intensity, duration, any associated symptoms, and the

CLUBBING OF THE FINGERS

normal 160°

Increased angle of the nail bed

IPD   DPD

Distal phalangeal depth (DPD) greater than the interphalangeal depth (IPD)

spongy

Softening of the nail bed

effect of any treatment or medications.

Next proceed with inspection, auscultation, palpation and percussion.

Begin with inspection

Look at the patient. Does he seem anxious or calm, tired or energetic? Does he seem to be in any distress?

Look for and ask about skin changes. Insufficient circulation can produce dry, brittle hair, dry skin with keratotic patches, and thickened nails (especially on the toes). Check for skin color:

• *Cyanosis* may indicate a congenital heart anomaly, congestive heart failure, or various pulmonary diseases. But keep in mind the difference between peripheral and central cyanosis. Peripheral cyanosis is on the finger tips and lips. It's not necessarily a sign of disease for you can see it in patients who are cold or anxious. Central cyanosis causes blue coloration on the mouth and lips, as well as the finger tips. It usually indicates a major oxygenation deficiency that accompanies heart and lung diseases.

• *Jaundice* occurs in late congestive heart failure and sometimes after heart surgery. It results from an increased bilirubin level. It's easiest to see in the sclerae.

• *Generalized pallor* can result from decreased levels of oxygenated hemoglobin (as in anemia). Pallor is often hard to evaluate because of individual variations in skin coloring. It's usually easiest to see in the conjunctivae, mouth, and nails.

Look for clubbing of the nails. It's common in patients with lung cancer, chronic obstructive lung disease, and congenital cardiovascular disease. To distinguish between normal familial roundness of the nails and clubbing, examine the angle between the nail bed and the finger. An angle greater than 160 degrees suggests clubbing (see insert).

Another sign of clubbing is an increase in the diameter of the fingertip that makes the distal phalangeal depth (DPD) greater than the interphalangeal depth (IPD). Also, watch for softening of the nail bed — a sign of chronic hypoxia.

Pay particular attention to venous distention or abnormal pulsation in the neck. It can indicate right-sided heart failure, right-sided valvular stenosis, pulmonary emboli, or cardiac tamponade. When assessing distention, use the internal jugular vein. Your reference point is the angle at which the manubrium fuses with the sternum (see insert). Record the estimated jugular venous distention as normal, increased, or markedly increased, along with the level of the head of the bed when you made the observation.

Proceed with inspection of the anterior chest in a systematic way. Concentrate on 5 areas: the aortic area, the second intercostal space to the right of the sternum; the pulmonic area, the second intercostal space to the left of the sternum; the right ventricular area, the lower half of the left sternal border; the apical area, the fifth intercostal space along the midclavicular line; and the epigastric area, near the xiphoid process. Carefully inspect each area for pulsations. Later you'll correlate these observations with other findings.

Palpation next

Feel the skin for temperature and moisture. Evaluate skin turgor by lifting a fold of the skin to see how promptly it returns to normal. Sluggish return to normal could mean dehydration. Also check for edema especially in the legs, sacrum, and other dependent areas. Press swollen areas with your fingers to see if indentations result (pitting edema).

Carefully assess all peripheral pulses. Include the carotids, brachials, radials, femorals, popliteals, dorsalis pedis, and posterior tibials. Note their rate, quality, and equality. They should be bilaterally equal. Rate the pulses on a scale of 0 to 4+. Zero is absent; 1+ is barely palpable; 2+ is normal or average; 3+ is full; 4+ is full, bounding, and often visible. (See insert, page 49, for the way they should test.)

When assessing arterial pulses you may find pulsus alternans. This is a variation in pulse in which weak impulses alternate with strong impulses. If you suspect pulsus alternans, apply a blood pressure cuff and elevate the pressure above the systolic level. Then gradually lower the pressure. At first you'll hear only the stronger beats. Then the pulse rate will double as the cuff pressure is lowered, and you'll hear weaker beats too. Pulsus alternans can indicate ventricular failure.

Another abnormal sign is a paradoxical pulse. Normally, the systolic blood pressure falls slightly (8 mm Hg) during inspiration. With paradoxical pulse, the fall is greater than 8 to 10 mm Hg. To detect it, apply a blood pressure cuff and raise the pressure to the systolic level so you hear beats only on expira-

Measuring the sternal angle
You can use the sternal angle to measure venous pressure and neck-vein distention. Here's how:

Elevate the head of the patient's bed to a 45° angle. Can you see venous pulsations in his neck? Do they rise above the sternal angle? In most cases, if the rise is no greater than 1 or 2 cm above the sternal angle, and if when the patient sits straight up the distention disappears, then his venous pressure falls within a normal range. However, if, when the patient sits straight up, you can still see venous distention, measure the highest point and alert the doctor. Venous distention like this may indicate heart failure, sometimes of the left side but more commonly of the right.

Aorta

Aortic
valve

Pulmonary
arteries

Pulmonary
veins

Pulmonary
valve

Left
atrium

Mitral
valve

Left
ventricle

Superior
vena
cava

Right
atrium

Tricuspid
valve

Right
ventricle

Inferior
vena
cava

Life's blood
This illustration shows the normal
circulation of blood through the
heart.

tion. Slowly deflate the cuff to the point where you hear impulses during both inspiration and expiration. The difference between the first reading and the second is the paradoxical pulse. It points to possible constrictive pericarditis or cardiac tamponade.

Palpate the chest in the same systematic way you used for inspection. In the same areas (aortic, pulmonic, right ventricular, apical, and epigastric), carefully palpate for pulsations or thrills (cat-purring vibrations). Use the ball of the hand to feel thrills; the finger pads to feel pulsations. If you find either, you'll have to correlate it with the heart sounds or with the carotid pulse.

In the apical area, pay special attention to the apical impulse. It's normally found in the fifth intercostal space at the left midclavicular line. This is usually called the point of maximal impulse (PMI). It correlates with ventricular systole and gives valuable information about abnormalities of the left ventricle. The PMI is usually only 1 to 2 cm in diameter, begins with the first heart sound, and lasts only to mid-systole. If it's larger or more lateral than normal, it could indicate left-sided valvular disease, coronary artery disease, or hypertension. If it's sustained and forceful, it could indicate left ventricular hypertrophy. You may detect left ventricular gallops in this same area. In patients with right ventricular pathology, the PMI may be found displaced to the right, closer to the sternum.

Percussion

Percussion will help you determine heart size. In the normal adult, the left cardiac border is near the point of maximal impulse, usually at or within the midclavicular line (MCL).

Percussion techniques used in examining the heart are the same as those for examining the lungs. With the patient lying down, begin to percuss his chest at the anterior axillary line. Start at the fifth intercostal space and move to the fourth, if necessary; percuss toward the sternum until you hear dullness. When you hear the change in the note, you have found the left border of cardiac dullness (LBCD). In the average adult male this is usually 10 to 12 cm from the midsternal line, and always within the midclavicular line. If the LBCD is greater than 12 cm from midsternum and outside the MCL, the heart may be enlarged. Only in a highly trained athlete can this be considered a normal finding.

If you have noticed anything abnormal so far, set out to confirm it through auscultation.

Auscultation

The key to successful auscultation is focusing on one sound at a time. Listen for *each of the four heart sounds at each location on the chest.* Before you can do this you must have a thorough grasp of the hemodynamic events that occur in the cardiac cycle. Review these events repeatedly until you know them well enough to identify each element of the cardiac cycle...when each valve opens and closes...systole and diastole.

For accurate auscultation, the stethoscope must be equipped with both a diaphragm (to hear higher pitched sounds) and a bell (to hear lower pitched sounds). Remember, the bell is effective only when placed on the chest wall very lightly.

Proceed with auscultation in a systematic, orderly fashion. Each heart valve and its related sounds are reflected to a specific area of the chest wall. You' and r the aortic valve sounds best in the second intercostal space to the right of the sternum; pulmonic sounds, in the second intercostal space to

Assessing peripheral pulses

Assess peripheral pulses bilaterally, noting their rate, quality, and equality. Here's how they should test:

	Right	Left
Temporal	2+	2+
Carotid	2+	2+
Brachial	2+	2+
Femoral	2+	2+
Popliteal	2+	2+
Posterior tibial	1+	1+
Dorsalis pedis	1+	1+

the left of the sternum; tricuspid sounds, in the fifth intercostal space near the left sternal border; and, mitral sounds in the fifth intercostal space near the midclavicular line. To be sure your auscultation is thorough, start at the aortic area and inch your way to each of the other valvular areas. Do this once with the diaphragm, and then once again using the bell.

S_1 — The first heart sound

At the beginning of ventricular systole, after the atria have been stimulated to contract, pressure rises in the ventricles to the point where it becomes higher than atrial pressure. At this point, the atrioventricular valves, the tricuspid on the right side and the mitral on the left side, are forced closed. As this occurs, the first heart sound or S_1 is transmitted to the chest wall. Since it results from closure of the mitral and tricuspid valves, this sound is normally loudest at the apex of the heart (around the fifth intercostal space at the left mid-clavicular line). Normally, the mitral valve closes slightly before the tricuspid valve but they are so close together that only one sound is heard. If for some reason the valve closure is separated, you can hear a splitting of S_1. When listening to S_1, listen carefully for intensity, consistency, and splitting.

S_2 — The second heart sound

As the cardiac cycle continues, after the atrioventricular valves close (S_1), the ventricle goes into the ejection phase of systole. This increased pressure forces open the semilunar valves, the pulmonic valve on the right side and the aortic valve on the left side. As systole ends and the ventricle starts to relax, there's a slight backflow of blood in the pulmonary artery and in the aorta. This backflow causes the pulmonic valve and the aortic valve to close. The sound transmitted to the chest wall at this time is the second heart sound (S_2). Since this sound results from closure of the pulmonic and aortic valves, S_2 is loudest at the base of the heart (the second intercostal space). Normally the aortic valve closes before the pulmonic valve, but so close together that only one sound is heard. If the valve closures separate, you can hear a splitting of S_2.

Listen to S_2, for intensity, consistency, and splitting. Since S_1 occurs at the beginning of systole and S_2 at the end of systole, the pause between S_1 and S_2 contains systolic sounds;

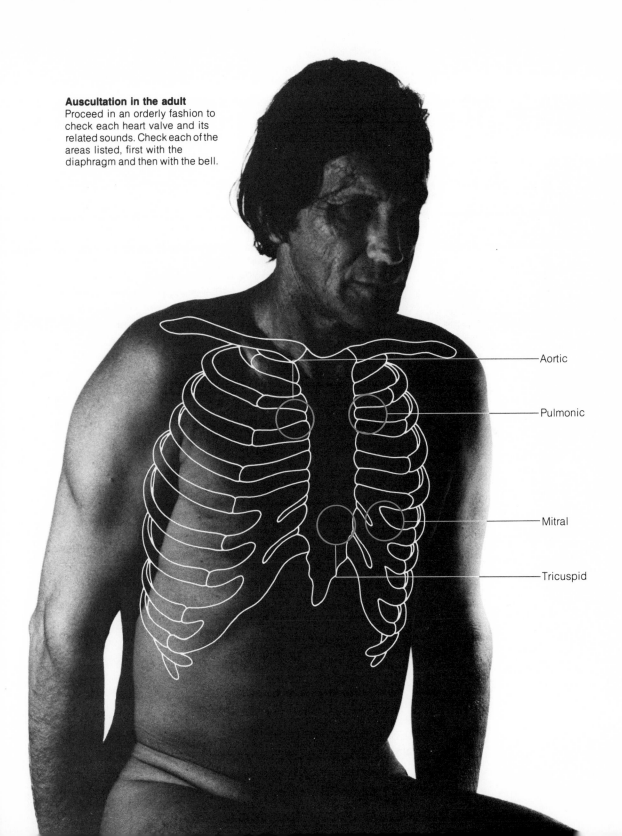

Auscultation in the adult
Proceed in an orderly fashion to
check each heart valve and its
related sounds. Check each of the
areas listed, first with the
diaphragm and then with the bell.

Aortic

Pulmonic

Mitral

Tricuspid

A full heart
The normal blood pressures and oxygen saturation levels in an adult heart are as follows:

SUPERIOR VENA CAVA (SVC)
Pressure — 2 to 14 mm Hg
             (maximum mean range)
             0 to 8 mm Hg
             (minimum mean range)
Oxygen — 70% to 87%

INFERIOR VENA CAVA (IVC)
Pressure — same as SVC
Oxygen — 77% to 85%

RIGHT ATRIUM (RA)
Pressure — $\dfrac{2 \text{ to } 14}{-2 \text{ to } +6}$ mm Hg
Oxygen — 74% to 86%

RIGHT VENTRICLE (RV)
Pressure — $\dfrac{15 \text{ to } 28}{0 \text{ to } 8}$ mm Hg
Oxygen — 71% to 87%

PULMONARY ARTERY (PA)
Pressure — $\dfrac{15 \text{ to } 28}{5 \text{ to } 16}$ mm Hg
Pulmonary wedge (PW)
Pressure — 6 to 15 mm Hg
                        (mean range)
Oxygen — 73% to 83%

LEFT ATRIUM (LA)
Pressure — $\dfrac{6 \text{ to } 20}{-2 \text{ to } +9}$ mm Hg
Oxygen — 94% to 100%

LEFT VENTRICLE (LV)
Pressure — $\dfrac{90 \text{ to } 140}{4 \text{ to } 12}$ mm Hg
Oxygen — 94% to 100%

the pause between S_2 and the next S_1 contains diastolic sounds.

S_3 — The third heart sound
The next event in the cardiac cycle is the resting phase of the ventricles (diastole). At the beginning of diastole, the pressure in the atria exceeds the pressure in the ventricles and causes the mitral and tricuspid valves to open. This allows a very rapid filling phase of the ventricles as the blood in the atria rushes into the ventricles. This sets up low frequency vibrations that are normally inaudible but you may detect them in some normal children and young adults, in patients with valvular regurgitation, or in those with ventricular failure. These low frequency sounds constitute the third heart sound or S_3. It's also called a diastolic filling sound or a ventricular gallop. It's heard best with the bell of the stethoscope when the patient lies in the left lateral position.

When S_3 results from left ventricular failure or aortic or mitral valvular regurgitation, it's heard best over the mitral area. If it results from right ventricular failure or right valvular regurgitation, it's heard best in the tricuspid area. Since an S_3 occurs at the beginning of diastole and a split S_2 occurs at the end of systole, you must listen carefully to distinguish between these two sounds.

S_4 — The fourth heart sound
Ventricular filling continues throughout diastole and ends with atrial contraction. This is a slow filling phase of the ventricle that creates low frequency sounds which, when audible, are the fourth heart sound or S_4. An S_4 is often found in patients with a decreased ventricular compliance (in hypertension, semilunar valvular stenosis, coronary artery disease, or an acute myocardial infarction). It's often heard in older patients, especially those over 65. It's also called a diastolic filling sound or an atrial gallop sound. Since it, too, is a low frequency sound, listen for it with the bell of the stethoscope (with the patient lying in left lateral position).

If S_4 results from left-sided dysfunction, you can hear it best in the mitral area; if from right-sided dysfunction, you can hear it best in the tricuspid area.

Since an S_4 occurs at the end of diastole and a split S_1 occurs at the beginning of systole, you must listen carefully to distin-

HOW VARIOUS KINDS OF CARDIAC PAIN DIFFER				
	ONSET AND DURATION	LOCATION AND RADIATION	QUALITY AND INTENSITY	SIGNS AND SYMPTOMS	PRECIPITATING FACTORS
MYOCARDIAL INFARCTION	Sudden onset; pain ½-2 hrs; residual soreness 1-3 days	Substernal, midline or anterior chest pain; radiation down one or both arms to jaw, neck, or back	Severe pressure; deep sensation: "crushing" "stabbing"	Apprehension, nausea, dyspnea, diaphoresis, increased blood pressure, gallop heart sound	Occurrence at rest or with exertion — physical or emotional
ANGINA	Gradual or sudden onset; pain usually lasts less than 15 min and not more than 30 min (average: 3 min)	Substernal or anterior chest pain, not sharply localized; radiation to back, neck, arms, jaw, even upper abdomen or fingers	Mild-to-moderate pressure, uniform pattern of attacks; deep sensation, tightness; "squeezing"	Dyspnea, diaphoresis, nausea, desire to void, belching, apprehension	Exertion, stress, eating, micturition or defecation; cold or hot, humid weather
PERICARDITIS	Sudden onset; continuous pain lasting for days; residual soreness	Substernal pain to left of midline; radiation to back or subclavicular area	Mild ache to severe pain, deep or superficial; "stabbing," "knife-like"	Precordial friction rub; increased pain with movement, inspiration, laughing, coughing, left side position; decreased pain with sitting or leaning forward (sitting up pulls the heart away from the diaphragm)	Myocardial infarction or upper respiratory infection; no relation to effort

guish these sounds, their location, pitch, timing, and duration.

Quadruple rhythm

Occasionally, you can hear both S_3 and an S_4 along with S_1 and S_2. This is called a quadruple rhythm. If this rhythm occurs in a patient whose pulse rate is faster than 110 beats per minute, the third and fourth heart sounds fuse to make one mid-diastolic sound. This is called a summation gallop.

Murmurs

Murmurs are sounds produced by abnormal turbulence. This turbulence can be caused by forward flow through a narrowed or irregular valve, or from backward flow through an incompetent valve. Murmurs are classified according to timing, intensity, location, pitch, quality, and radiation.

When timing a murmur, you must establish if it occurs during diastole or during systole. Remember if you hear a murmur between S_1 and S_2, it's a systolic murmur; between S_2 and the next S_1, it's a diastolic murmur. Fine timing is deciding exactly where in systole or in diastole the murmur occurs — for example, mid-diastole or late systole.

Grade the intensity of the murmur from I to VI. Grade I is very faint; II is soft and low; III is prominent but not palpable; IV is prominent and palpable (you can feel a thrill); V is very loud; and Grade VI is audible with the stethoscope off the chest.

Murmurs that occur during systole (because of left-sided pathology) are the murmurs of aortic stenosis and mitral regurgitation. Those that occur during systole (because of right-sided pathology) are the murmurs of pulmonic stenosis and tricuspid regurgitation. Murmurs that occur during diastole (when the left ventricle is filling) are the murmurs of mitral stenosis and aortic regurgitation. Murmurs that occur during diastole (when the right ventricle is filling) are the murmurs of tricuspid stenosis and pulmonic regurgitation.

Each of these eight murmurs has unique characteristics of timing, quality, location, pitch, and radiation. Beginners at auscultation should first classify these murmurs according to timing, location, and intensity. Only with experience can you learn to recognize the other more subtle characteristics.

Pericardial friction rub

In patients who have pericarditis, you may hear a pericardial friction rub. This is a high-pitched, scratchy sound that seems close to the listener's ear. It can have three components: atrial systole; ventricular systole; and ventricular diastole. You can hear a pericardial friction rub best with the diaphragm of the stethoscope when the patient leans forward. The sound comes and goes without any discernible pattern. It's usually located around the fourth or fifth intercostal space from the sternal border to the apex.

Your patients with cardiovascular problems need frequent assessment so that your nursing interventions correspond to their changing condition. If you can examine a chest competently, you can give them this kind of care. But don't be discouraged if you don't learn the whole approach at once. Such competence takes a lot of patients...and patience.

Diagnostic Tests
Invasive and noninvasive

BY ARLENE B. STRONG, RN, MN

DEFINING A PATIENT'S CARDIOVASCULAR problems often depends on the results of certain diagnostic tests and procedures. While you do not usually order these tests or do them, you do need to know what they are so you can prepare the patient for them both physically and psychologically. To do this you must know why a certain test is apt to be ordered, and what the patient can expect during the procedure and afterward so you can consider these things when planning the patient's care.

Here are the tests and procedures most commonly used in identifying cardiovascular disease and what you need to know about them.

Noninvasive tests first

Chest X-rays are usually among the first tests ordered when there is any reason to suspect myocardial malfunction. They are used primarily to show cardiac enlargement and pulmonary congestion. X-rays can show *pulmonary congestion* resulting from left heart failure as an opacity in the central hilar region that fans out peripherally from the hilar region and gives the area above the base of the heart the look of "antlers."

In chronic forms of pulmonary hypertension, you may see

On the lookout
Conditions such as congestive heart failure and pulmonary edema can be diagnosed and evaluated with chest X-rays like the one above. Here you can see hilar congestion and prominent pulmonary vascular markings. These "butterfly or bat-wing configurations," as they are sometimes called, indicate congestion. Notice, too, how enlarged the patient's heart is.

interstitial edema as diffuse cloudiness in the central lung fields that may resemble the shape of a butterfly. You may also notice blunting of the costophrenic angles that reflects fluid accumulation in these interlobular spaces. If a great deal of fluid accumulates, you may see marked opaque lines at the periphery or even more centrally (Kerley B or Kerley A lines). These chest X-rays findings can detect interstitial edema even before auscultatory findings become abnormal.

Alveolar edema appears as "cotton-puff" cloudiness in the central lung field that spreads peripherally and superiorly as edema in the air sacs worsens. Such accumulations of fluid produce fine mid- to late inspiratory rales. X-ray confirms the auscultatory findings and helps determine the extent of the edema.

You can detect *cardiac enlargement* on chest X-rays by estimating the cardiothoracic ratio. To get a fairly accurate estimate, measure the diameter of the cardiac silhouette at its widest point; then compare it to the widest diameter of the thoracic cage. The thoracic cage should be at least twice as wide as the heart (except on posterior-anterior [P-A] views taken by portable X-ray). Of course, comparison with previous X-rays can greatly help in evaluating cardiac size, especially in patients with chronic lung disease. Such a patient's heart may be quite small compared to that in a person with normal lungs. What is cardiac enlargement for one may be within the "normal" limits for others.

When comparing chest X-rays for cardiac enlargement, be sure to note whether the X-ray was taken during maximum inspiration. To get the most information from chest X-rays, motivate the patient to take the deepest breath he can during this test. If the patient is lethargic or confused, you may have to call on a family member to persuade the patient to cooperate.

Standard chest X-rays are usually taken with the patient standing upright. However, if the patient is unable to stand, chest X-rays may be taken at the bedside. When preparing a patient for bedside X-ray, be sure to elevate the head of the bed as high as the patient can tolerate. This reduces the pressure of the abdominal contents on the diaphragm and, consequently, on the thoracic structures and allows a better X-ray.

Chest X-rays may also show *cardiac calcifications*. However, in order to determine their exact location (valvular or subvalvular), additional tests are required.

Fluoroscopic and other tests

The cardiac fluoroscopic examination allows the examiner to see the heart from different views while it is in motion. For example, fluoroscopy of cardiac calcifications and their motion during the cardiac cycle helps to pinpoint their location. Cardiac fluoroscopy helps to evaluate wall motion and movement of prosthetic heart valves. It also identifies ventricular aneurysm (a paradoxical bulging motion of the aneurysmal sac appears during cardiac systole).

The *cardiac series* is a fluoroscopic cardiac examination in which the examiner watches the descent of swallowed barium through the esophagus from different angles. Since the esophagus is anatomically located immediately behind the heart, cardiac enlargement changes esophageal contour. Cardiac fluoroscopic examinations are given in an upright position; unlike the gastrointestinal series, they don't require the patient to fast beforehand. Many institutions avoid using fluoroscopy because it entails increased exposure to radiation. They concentrate instead on more benign techniques — usually echocardiography and electrocardiography.

Echocardiography uses ultrasound to study the location and motion of heart structures. A transducer, the size of a dime, is placed on the sternum with the tip directed towards the structures being studied. Then, ultrahigh frequency sound waves of short duration are transmitted through the transducer to these structures. The same transducer receives the echos produced as the sound waves reverberate; in turn, it relays the echos to the echocardiograph machine which records these sounds on paper.

The echos produced this way vary with the density and mobility of the structures. A trained interpreter can examine recorded echos and conclude from them information about valve leaflet mobility and position, heart wall motion during systole and diastole, and any extraneous "noises" that may be coming from intracardiac growths. Echocardiography has proven especially valuable for diagnosing atrial myxomas, ventricular aneurysms and pericardial effusions. It's also used for assessing mitral and aortic valvular dysfunction, cardiac chamber dilatation, myocardial hypertrophy, and abnormal septal wall motion.

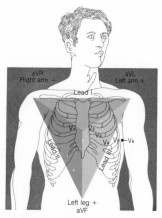

The 12-lead EKG
The 12-lead EKG uses electrodes to picture different anatomical areas of the heart and to pinpoint sites of damage.
There are 3 groups of leads:
• *Standard limb leads* (I, II, III) These bipolar leads (2 electrodes) simultaneously record the electrical forces of the heart as they flow toward the extremities. The right arm is always the negative pole; the left leg always positive. The left arm can be positive (in lead I) or negative (in lead III). When current flows toward the positive pole, the deflections of the EKG wave will be upright. When it flows toward the negative pole, the deflections will be inverted.
• *Unipolar augmented leads* record activity from the shoulders and the left leg and are called aVR (augmented right), aVL (augmented left), and aVF (augmented foot).
• *Precordial leads* (V_1 to V_6) record the electrical activity from 6 different positions on the chart. They are designed by the letter V and a number.

How to prepare patients for echocardiography? Mainly, relieve their anxiety about this relatively unfamiliar procedure. Patients might expect needles, electric charges, or X-rays, but echocardiography is a painless and benign procedure. The patient merely lies flat on his back or on his left side for about 15 minutes. During this time, he may be asked to breathe in certain ways to help direct the sound waves toward the heart structures being studied.

Sometimes echocardiography and phonocardiography are combined in a procedure called echophonocardiography. This makes it possible to compare cardiac motion (obtained by echocardiograph) and the recorded cardiac sounds. It can identify the position of the valves and aortic valve leaflets during abnormal heart sounds and thus pinpoint the source of abnormal sounds. Your patient should know that during the echophonocardiography, a trained observer will be listening to his amplified heart sounds. The room must be very quiet to eliminate the recording of extraneous sounds. Just as during echocardiography, the patient may be asked to turn, lie flat, or perform specific breathing maneuvers.

EKG indispensable

Cardiovascular evaluation is incomplete without a 12-lead electrocardiogram (EKG). This graphic display of cardiac electrical activity provides invaluable data. It's one of the few diagnostic tests that you may be responsible for doing and must know how to interpret outside of an intensive care setting. To do this, you need to know the normal cardiac electrical events, including conduction and recording (see insert).

The 12-lead EKG records electrical activity from 12 universally accepted lead placements and offers a comprehensive assessment of cardiac electrical events. The 12-lead EKG offers much more information than the single lead commonly used for intensive care monitoring. Quite typically, deviations from normal occur in some leads, and not in others. If you're shopping for a car, you don't inspect it from one angle. You walk all around it. Just so, the 12-lead EKG "walks" around the heart to record its electrical phenomena from different angles.

Remember, though, that some abnormalities occur only intermittently (such as arrhythmias or ischemic disturbances). The standard 12-lead EKG records only about 70 electrical impulses out of more than 100,000 that occur in 24 hours. So, understandably, intermittent abnormalities are easily missed. Moreover, an EKG disturbance may show only when the patient has symptoms (which he may perceive as outright pain or as vague discomfort), or during exercise. For this reason, a doctor may order a 12-lead EKG to be done during an episode of chest pain (when repolarization disturbances from cardiac ischemia are most likely to show). Ischemic chest pain produces a depression in the S-T segment, an inversion of the T wave, or both S-T segment and T wave deviations. When chest pain subsides the EKG usually reverts to normal. So if you're testing a patient during chest pain, be sure to complete the test before giving drugs such as nitroglycerin to relieve it. Obviously, you must complete it as quickly as possible so the patient doesn't have to endure the pain any longer than necessary. Be sure to mark the tracing as one taken during chest pain.

Who needs an EKG?

Ideally, every adult should have a baseline 12-lead EKG, once every 5 years. Obviously an EKG is indicated for diagnosis of acute myocardial infarction and throughout recovery from it. An EKG is also useful whenever there's any reason to expect changes from previous recordings; for monitoring electrolyte abnormalities; or monitoring the effects of drugs that influence cardiac electrical function.

The stress test (EKG during exercise) is one of the best noninvasive tools for assessing cardiac response to increased workload. This test has proven value for determining functional capacity after heart surgery and, after myocardial infarction (at least 14 days after the acute event), to establish readiness for an exercise program. It's also used to identify cardiac ischemia as the source of chest discomfort. The exercise test does not require that your patient fast. However, he should not have food, cigarettes, or caffeinated beverages for 2 hours before the test.

The exercise test can be done on a special bicycle (on which the workload can be set and increased) or on treadmills with adjustable speed and grade controls. Throughout this test, the cardiogram is continuously monitored along with occasional simultaneous recordings of the patient's blood pressure response. Throughout, the patient is asked about any symptoms.

Making waves

The waves of an EKG correlate with the electrical stimulation that precedes the mechanical contraction and relaxation of the heart. These waves have arbitrarily been labeled the P, QRS, and T waves.

The P wave reflects depolarization of the atria, and therefore is a good indication of SA node function. The QRS complex reflects the depolarization of the ventricles. The T wave reflects the repolarization of the ventricles. (The T wave corresponding to the repolarization of the atria isn't visible, as the QRS deflection obscures it.) The mass of the ventricles is much greater than that of the atria, so the QRS and T waves are much larger than the P wave.

Occasionally, another wave called a U wave will appear after the T wave.

Heart blocks
In reading 12-lead EKGs, remember that the vertical lines measure the magnitude of the electrical impulse of the heart. The horizontal lines represent the time the electrical impulse takes to travel over cardiac tissue. Each small block on EKG paper is 1 mm tall and 0.04 seconds wide.

The test ends at the discretion of the doctor in attendance. Indications for termination of the test include any of the following: extreme fatigue, onset of angina for which the patient would normally stop activity, a drop in blood pressure, onset of arrhythmia, significant S-T changes, or attainment of desired heart rate without abnormal findings. The latter constitutes a negative test.

What constitutes a positive stress test? The criteria vary. Some institutions require S-T segment depression of 1.5 to 2 mm. In about 15% of the patients with *positive tests,* coronary artery disease cannot be documented by invasive diagnostic studies. In 15% of the patients with *negative tests,* coronary arteriography shows definite coronary artery disease. False positives may result from: digitalis, hypertension, or electrolyte abnormalities. If the patient is unable (because of drugs or fatigue) to exercise sufficiently to raise the heart rate to the point of stress, the test is considered nondiagnostic.

What are the contraindications for stress testing? Any recent history of unusually long or severe episodes of angina, chest pain with dyspnea, weakness, diaphoresis, nausea or vomiting. Always check with the doctor before beginning an exercise test in a patient with any of these symptoms.

Who needs the stress test? Some doctors believe everyone over 35 should have this test every 2 years. Others feel that it's indicated only for patients suspected of having ischemic heart disease. Lately, many centers are using the exercise test to determine physical fitness and to prescribe individual exercise programs.

Three invasive tests
1. *Myocardial imaging* uses radioactive tracers to evaluate cardiac structures and function much the same as they are used for testing brain, liver, and other structures. Radioactive tracers are nontoxic substances such as albumin or potassium which can be labeled with a radioactive substance and easily carried by the blood stream. Their course through the body can then be followed and recorded by scanners.

In some tests, an absence of tracer material ("cold spots") indicates decreased perfusion. In other tests, increased uptake of tracer material ("hot spots"), indicates greater than normal perfusion. Such perfusion studies can help identify acute myocardial infarction by detecting defects in myocardial perfusion or regional myocardial wall abnormalities. They can also be used to screen asymptomatic patients who have a positive stress test. Such patients are scanned during rest and during exercise. The test results are then compared. Radioactive tracer studies can also evaluate ventricular function. As the tracer passes through the heart chambers, it can show heart wall motion, chamber size and shape, and the percentage of blood ejected. The patient undergoing radioactive tracer evaluation needs an intravenous infusion to carry the tracer material. Be sure to tell him that the amount of radioactivity used is extremely small and not harmful to himself or those near him. He needs no special care after this test.

2. *Cardiac enzymes* are intracellular substances used during metabolism. Injury to the cell membrane such as occurs during an acute myocardial infarction releases these enzymes from the cell into the blood stream. To detect these enzymes, it's important to draw the blood sample for the test as soon after the injury as possible (see Chapter 8).

3. *Cardiac catheterization* has become a fairly common procedure for confirming a diagnosis, assessing the severity of cardiac abnormality, or evaluating a condition for surgery. You should know what's involved in performing catheterization studies, what the test results mean, and how to assess and handle possible postprocedure complications.

Preparing your patient

A patient entering a cath lab for the first time can become apprehensive unless prepared for the experience. The lab contains an overwhelming array of machinery: motion picture cameras, a fluoroscope, one or more electrocardiographs, pressure-monitoring devices, and numerous other paraphernalia. To prepare your patient, tell him that he'll be placed on a special X-ray table, virtually surrounded by equipment, some of which is even suspended from the ceiling. Once he's settled with EKG leads attached, he'll have an antecubital fossa or the groin prepped for catheter insertion. These are the sites doctors most commonly use. Sometimes, they use the axillary artery through a puncture site a few inches below the armpit. At times, the first attempt at catheter insertion is unsuccessful, because of an anatomical abnormality or blockage within the target vessel. Then a second site must be used.

During the catheterization, your patient may be asked to

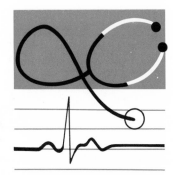

Common assessment tests for cardiac malfunction

MUSCLE DYSFUNCTION
 chest roentgenography
 resting 12-lead EKG
 stress test
 echocardiography
 echophonocardiography
 cardiac angiography

VALVULAR MALFUNCTION
 chest roentgenography
 resting 12-lead EKG
 echocardiography
 echophonocardiography
 cardiac angiography

ELECTRICAL ABNORMALITIES
 resting 12-lead EKG
 24-hour Holter monitoring
 stress test

CORONARY ARTERY DISEASE
 resting 12-lead EKG
 24-hour Holter monitoring
 stress test
 coronary angiography-
  arteriography
 cardiac enzyme studies

cough or to take deep breaths. You can tell him why. Deep-breathing can facilitate catheter placement into the coronary arteries, pulmonary artery, or the wedge position. And coughing may counteract the nausea, light-headedness or initial hypotension that sometimes follows the injection of contrast medium (dye). Be sure your patient knows how to cough; he must do it correctly and as soon as he is told. But, if hypotension persists, the patient may need treatment with a pressor agent. So during catheterization, monitor constantly for arrhythmias and for changes in blood pressure. Also, keep handy the equipment you need for CPR and defibrillation.

Cardiac cathereterization is especially helpful in evaluating....

• *Valvular efficiency.* Pressure measurements in the pulmonary artery and pulmonary capillary wedge positions provide information about pressure in the left atrium and, in many instances, the left ventricle. Mitral valve disease will elevate pressures in the left atrium, hampering blood flow from the pulmonary vessels. Pressure in the pulmonary vessels (particularly the veins and capillaries) then rises to compensate for the higher atrial pressure (pulmonary hypertension).

If your patient has *mitral valve* disease, he may be asked to exercise (pedaling leg motion) during catheterization to increase venous return to his heart. The greater the degree of mitral disease, the higher the pressure in the pulmonary capillaries during exercise, as compared with the resting pressure (which may be normal).

• *Stenosis.* Systolic pressure measurements, made on both sides of a *stenotic aortic valve,* will show a difference (or gradient) across the valve. The higher the gradient, the greater the stenosis. For example, left ventricular systolic pressure might measure 200 mm Hg and aortic systolic pressure only 120 mm Hg. That's an 80 mm Hg gradient across the valve. Since these pressures normally are equal, a stenosis that makes this big a difference usually requires corrective surgery.

• *Septal defects.* These defects can be evaluated by measuring blood oxygen content on each side of the abnormal septum. Elevated blood oxygen on the right indicates a left-to-right shunt at either the atrial or ventricular level. A decreased oxygen on the left indicates a right-to-left shunt.

• *Myocardial function.* Injection of contrast medium into the

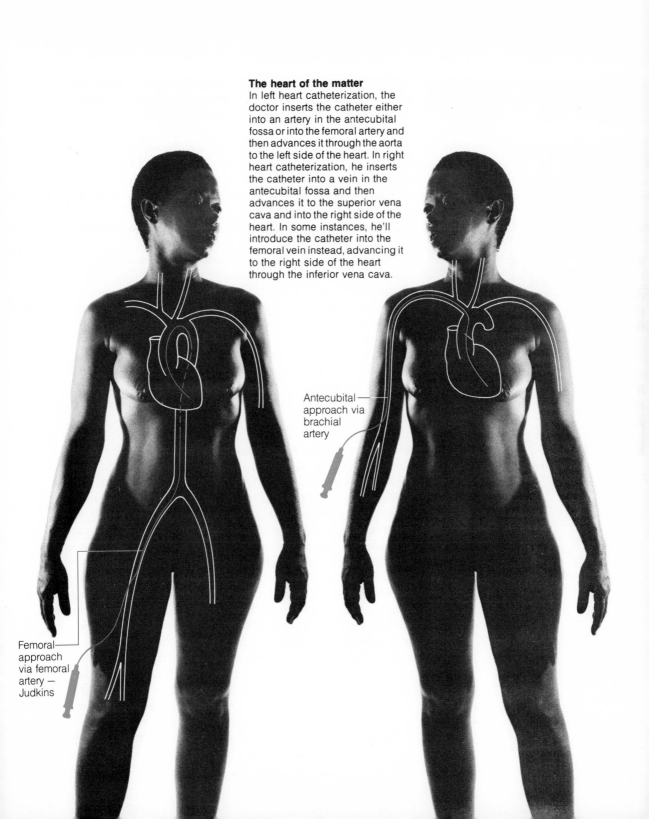

The heart of the matter
In left heart catheterization, the doctor inserts the catheter either into an artery in the antecubital fossa or into the femoral artery and then advances it through the aorta to the left side of the heart. In right heart catheterization, he inserts the catheter into a vein in the antecubital fossa and then advances it to the superior vena cava and into the right side of the heart. In some instances, he'll introduce the catheter into the femoral vein instead, advancing it to the right side of the heart through the inferior vena cava.

Antecubital approach via brachial artery

Femoral approach via femoral artery — Judkins

State of the heart
Cardiac catheterization includes two procedures: coronary arteriography and coronary ventriculography. For the first procedure, the patient is placed in the right anterior oblique (RAO) position. Contrast medium or dye is injected into the left coronary artery, as in figure 1. As you can see, the vessel fills completely, without narrowing or occlusion.

For ventriculography, the patient is again placed in the RAO position. During diastole, contrast medium is injected into the left ventricle. The picture that results shows wall motion, ventricular volume, the shape of the left ventricle, and the presence of any mechanical abnormalities. Figure 2 shows a normal left ventricle.

left ventricle (ventriculography) is used to assess structure and contractility of the cardiac muscle. Comparison of ventricular size during systole and diastole helps determine efficiency of muscular contraction, segmental wall motion, chamber size, and ejection fraction. The latter compares the amount of blood pumped out of the left ventricle during systole and the amount remaining at the end of diastole. For example, at rest, the normal left ventricle contains about 100 ml of blood. If the ventricle ejects 70 ml during systole, the ejection fraction is 70/100 (70%). In myocardial incompetency, the ejection fraction is less than 55%.

• *Wall motion.* Improper contraction of a portion of the heart chamber wall, called wall motion abnormality, commonly develops after myocardial infarction. Such a defect is called hypokinesis (reduced wall motion), akinesis (absence of motion), or dyskinesis (bulging in the wall during a systole).

How is this test done? Using the Sones or Judkins technique, the doctor threads a catheter (visually controlled with fluoroscopy) through an artery and advances it to the aortic root and passes it across the aortic valve into the left ventricle. He then injects contrast medium (an opaque dye) into this area.

Arteriography: Coronary road map

Coronary arteriography, an important part of the cardiac catheterization test, produces a radiographic study of the arteries that supply the myocardium. With coronary arteriography the doctor can see the coronary arteries as clearly as you see a superhighway on a road map. Arteriography shows the sites, degree, and severity of obstruction in the coronary vessels. It allows evaluation of the size, character of blood flow and the presence of atherosclerotic disease of vessels distal to the obstruction. This is an important factor in determining whether the vessel can be bypassed. So, coronary arteriograms are often used to determine if a patient can benefit from surgery. Candidates for coronary bypass graft surgery must have significant lesions that can actually be bypassed. They can't be if the disease is too diffuse, or if the vessel is too small to accept a graft. During evaluation for bypass, patients often receive nitroglycerin to augment left ventricular contractility and thus show if potential revascularization will be beneficial.

Coronary arteriography requires moving the patient from

side to side so the stationary camera (suspended from the ceiling) directly over the patient can record views of the coronary vessels from different angles. Warn the patient that he will be asked to move. Two common positions he'll be asked to assume are the right anterior oblique (RAO) and the left anterior oblique (LAO). When the patient is in RAO position, the doctor can view and film the anterior basal, anterior, apical and inferior walls and vessels of the myocardium as well as the basal wall segment of the left ventricle. The LAO position shows the septum and posterior laterial wall of the myocardium.

Warn the patient to expect a feeling of flushing and warmth as the dye is injected. This is normal. Assure the patient that if he develops chest pain during the procedure, he'll receive nitroglycerin to relieve it. Tell him what other symptoms he may experience during the procedure. Explain that, before he goes to the cath lab, he'll have a sedative to help him relax. But it won't put him to sleep, because his cooperation will be needed during the test procedure (taking deep breaths, turning, and so forth). Remember that your reassurance and understanding are essential to allay any fear the patient may have.

Watch for complications

Severe complications after cardiac catheterization are not common, but can occur. The period of greatest danger is during the procedure itself when complications such as arterial occlusion from embolus, arterial spasm, AMI, or perforation of the myocardium can occur. Watch for: isolated premature ventricular contractions, ventricular tachycardia and ventricular fibrillation, which can occur during or after the procedure.

If a thrombus breaks loose, or if a plaque dislodges, it can block the patient's blood flow. Rarely, he may suffer a cerebrovascular accident or myocardial infarction. If the blocked vessel is an artery, your patient can lose his arterial pulse. Then the extremity itself will be white and cold. Your patient may complain of a numb feeling or severe pain.

Blood loss at the catheter insertion site is usually more profuse from arteriotomies than venotomies. If you see frank bleeding or notice swelling of the extremity at the insertion site, apply pressure to the site. The amount of pressure you apply must be greater than the pressure in the vessel. In the case of an artery, for example, the pressure applied must be greater than the systolic pressure at that site. Anytime significant bleeding occurs, whether venous or arterial, your patient's pressure will drop and his heart rate will increase. Watch for such bleeding, since even slight leakage into surrounding tissues can cause a painful hematoma. Infection at the site is another potential complication. To prevent it, keep the area clean and dry. Use aseptic technique when caring for the site or changing the dressing.

After catheterization

Take vital signs frequently, as often as every 10 to 15 minutes and record them on the patient's chart. Include blood pressure, heart rate, and pulse distal to the catheter insertion site. When checking blood pressure, make certain not to wrap the cuff on the arm that was used for arterial puncture because this increases the risk of hemorrhage or arterial occlusion. When you take vital signs, check the pressure dressing over the insertion site(s). Check to be sure dressings are dry and intact, but not too tight. Then examine the extremity distal to the insertion site for color and warmth, and assess the quality of its pulse. Your patient will need about 6 hours of strict bedrest immediately after the test. During that time, remind him to keep the extremity straight since bending will loosen the dressing and may cause bleeding. This is particularly important when the patient is moved from the stretcher to the bed. During this move, make sure you apply pressure to the site, especially if the Judkins technique (femoral insertion) was used. The patient can usually resume bending his arm or leg about 6 hours after the test. Before that, he should wiggle his fingers or toes every half hour. Tell the patient that if he has pain when the local anesthetic wears off, he can have an analgesic.

You can do much to help patients through cardiac catheterization and other tests if you understand the tests yourself, know what their effects can be, and take the time to tell patients what to expect.

Hypertension
Risk factor in atherosclerosis

BY ROSEMARY JARLATH MALONEY, BSN, MSN

IF YOU MANAGE hypertensive patients at all, you know that the worst problem is getting them to stick to their prescribed regimen. They typically miss appointments, forget to take their medications, and neglect their diet. If they'd only cooperate, they would be much better off and you could feel better about their treatment. All too often they don't. Some sources suggest that only 13% of hypertensive patients seem to be under good control.

How can you help?

Often, patients with hypertension don't cooperate because they don't understand how hypertension is threatening their lives. You can help them to understand. First, you must understand hypertension quite well yourself.

What is hypertension? The American Heart Association, recognizing that it's different things in different people, simply calls it an *unstable or persistent elevation of pressure above the normal range.* And they estimate that more than 26 million people in the U.S. and Canada suffer from it. *That's one in every six adults.*

The prevalence among women is 3% to 4% higher than

Probable causes of hypertension

According to 1978 estimates of the American Heart Association, among people 20 years old and over, 13% of white males and 25% of black males, 17% of white females and 28% of black females have hypertension. Hypertension may be a primary or secondary disorder. This chart shows you at a glance the diagnostic possibilities according to age of onset. For example, you can see that as a person ages, the possibility of developing renal parenchymal disease or aortic coarctation decreases while the possibility of developing primary aldosteronism or essential hypertension increases. People of all ages are susceptible to pheochromocytoma.
Understanding these trends will help you assess your patient.

- ■ ■ Renal arterial disease
- ⟍⟍⟍ Renal parenchymal disease
- ■■■ Aortic coarctation
- ▬▬▬ Pheochromocytoma
- ■ ■ Essential hypertension
- ⟍▬⟍ Primary aldosteronism

PROBABLE · POSSIBLE · IMPROBABLE

Up to 20 years old   20 to 35 years old

among men; among blacks, 11% to 12% higher than among whites (see above). Target organs — those chiefly affected — are brain, eyes, heart, and kidneys. Early symptoms? Typically, there aren't any. Or the victim may have morning headache. But the damage can go on just the same as the pressure rises.

Why blood pressure varies

Blood pressure is the relationship between a given amount and flow of fluid, the blood, and the size and tension of its container, the vessel walls. Its purpose, of course, is to perfuse even the remotest tissue with life-giving oxygen carried by the circulating red blood cells. But there are numerous variables in the two factors, blood flow and vasculature. Hence the variations in pressure.

Variables are these. The quantity of blood flow in a given time, cardiac output, is determined by: ventricular filling (partly based on plasma volume); the heart's contractility; the heart rate (primarily controlled by the autonomic nervous system); and, total peripheral vascular resistance. Peripheral vascular resistance itself depends on the caliber and tone of the

35 to 50 years old   50 years old and over

arteries, arterioles, and veins. Unless the vessels are largely
occluded by atherosclerosis or some other mechanical blockage, their capacity is powerfully regulated by humoral and
neural stimulation also coming from the autonomic nervous
system.

Humoral agents, such as angiotensin, catecholamines,
serotonin, histamine, prostaglandins, and aldosterone influence the size of the blood vessels and blood volume (by
regulating sodium and water balance). Neural control is even
quicker and more efficient; witness the "fight or flight" reaction to stress.

Hypertension can be controlled by manipulating almost any
one of these factors, as modern pharmacological agents do.
First, though, you must know what's causing it.

Classification of hypertension falls into essential and secondary. *Essential* hypertension — about 80% to 90% of all
cases — has no proven cause. One theory says it's caused by
increased peripheral vascular resistance coming from degenerative constriction of the arterioles. This resistance produces renal ischemia which, in turn, stimulates the renin-
angiotensin and aldosterone cycles.

What meets the eye
This eye ground, of a 43-year-old woman, shows Grade III changes in the retina. The patient had malignant hypertension, blurred vision, papilledema of the left disc, fresh hemorrhage, and impending vein occlusion.

The remaining cases of hypertension stem from a secondary cause: renal vascular stenosis or occlusion, for example, or renal parenchymal disease, pheochromocytoma or some other endocrine disturbance, coarctation of the aorta, or toxemia of pregnancy. Primary aldosteronism is another secondary cause. It produces hypervolemia by inducing an excess reabsorption of sodium and water. Lately, another cause has been found — the use of oral contraceptives.

Although hypertension can occur at any age, even in childhood, essential hypertension usually occurs between the ages of 30 and 50. Contributing factors? Often, obesity, a high sodium intake, and elevated cholesterol and triglyceride levels. And familial predisposition: Siblings of known hypertensives have an added susceptibility to it.

The role of stress? Because stress, anger, and frustration momentarily drive the blood pressure up, stress has been implicated as a principal factor in keeping it there. The problem is, eventually relieving the stress doesn't usually bring the blood pressure down. But, indeed, implicating stress are these facts: Black men in high-stress situations have higher incidence of hypertension than any other group; people in societies undergoing change have a higher incidence than those in stable populations. Although arterial pressure tends to increase with advancing age in most societies, studies of Pacific island natives and Brazilian Indians have shown that such people escape hypertension as a natural consequence of age.

Diagnostic clues
You can often assess a patient's cardiovascular status by whether he has dyspnea, orthopnea, or chest pain. Dependent edema would indicate failure of cardiac venous return, probably from right-sided heart failure. Nocturia could mean kidney involvement or heart failure. Nocturia occurs as a result of recumbency at night (increased perfusion of the renal bed enhances filtration and excretion).

If he has nephrosclerosis along with hypertension, proteinuria would result from the increased renal arteriolar permeability. Uremia is seldom seen in benign essential hypertension, but it is one of the hallmarks of the relentless, progressive form known as malignant hypertension. Papilledema is pathognomonic of malignant hypertension, and it's often accompanied by renal and cerebral symptoms. In benign essential hypertension, the early morning headache often reported in the beginning may be succeeded by fatigue, diminished mental acuity, forgetfulness, and irritability, brought on by "small strokes" — minor cerebrovascular accidents.

Examining the optic fundi gives perhaps the best information about the severity and duration of the hypertensive process. Usually, mild hypertensive retinopathy can be seen as constriction of the vessels of the eyegrounds. If you see soft exudates, hemorrhages, and papilledema, they lend an ominous prognosis. End-stage retinopathy is reflected by venous destruction and arterial obliteration, that is, the vessels thicken enough to close the intimal lumen. Unfortunately, these arteriosclerotic changes are irreversible.

Cardiac disease itself can either produce or result from the hypertensive process. Either way, cardiac involvement is the leading cause of death in hypertensive patients. So, assessment in hypertensive patients always includes thorough auscultation for changes in heart sounds (see Chapter 4).

Lab work should include some or all of these tests:

• Chest film to show cardiac size and pulmonary vasculature.

• Blood urea nitrogen (BUN) and serum creatinine to measure renal excretory function.

• Protein excretion in the urine measured over a 24-hour period, which shouldn't total more than 0.2 to 0.4 gram; if higher, it indicates renal parenchymal disease.

• Serum electrolytes, especially potassium levels (which inversely denote the secretory levels of aldosterone) since that hormone saves sodium by wasting potassium and hydrogen ions in the renal tubule.

• EKG to check for left ventricular hypertrophy characteristic of hypertensive heart disease.

Treatment goals

Treatment of hypertension aims to reduce arterial pressure and arrest atherosclerosis and progressive arteriolar disease. Most doctors consider cardiovascular risk reduced when diastolic readings are maintained at less than 90 mm Hg. This can be accomplished in up to 85% of patients.

Three kinds of drugs are used to lower blood pressure:

1. Diuretics act by promoting water and sodium excretion,

What is hypertensive crisis?

An acute rise in blood pressure (diastolic usually over 120 mm Hg). Thickening and narrowing of arterioles lead to damage of vital organs. *What precipitates it* in some hypertensive patients?

• abrupt discontinuation of antihypertensive medications
• increased salt consumption
• increased production of renin, epinephrine, and norepinephrine
• increased stress.

Therapy aims:
To lower blood pressure rapidly to prevent hypertensive encephalopathy by use of vasodilators, I.V. (nitroprusside, diazoxide, hydralazine) and sympathetic blockers (methyldopa, phentolamine, reserpine). Trimethaphan camsylate blocks both sympathetic and parasympathetic nervous systems.

Nursing responsibilities:
• Take baseline vital signs and monitor frequently: blood pressure readings from both arms, apical pulse, respirations, and temperature. Check pupils for reaction to light; assess level of consciousness and orientation to time, place, person.
• Check for dehydration. Remember, giving vasodilators to dehydrated patients can cause dangerous hypotension.
• Obtain a patient history.
• Be supportive to patient and family.
• Monitor drug therapy to prevent severe hypotension or toxic reactions.
• Teach patient and family as soon as possible about: drugs, diet, activities, avoidance of stress, and how to take home blood pressures.

Secondary hypertension

The following disorders can cause secondary hypertension, so watch for the physical findings that accompany each.

COARCTATION OF AORTA — absence of femoral pulses, decreased blood pressure in legs, weight loss, intercostal bruits.

PHEOCHROMOCYTOMA — severe headache with palpitation, hypermetabolic state, elevated fasting blood sugar.

PRIMARY ALDOSTERONISM — elevated blood pressure, weakness, nocturia, polydipsia, tetany, headache, numbness, hypokalemia.

CUSHING'S SYNDROME — moon face, "buffalo" hump, edema.

VASCULAR RENAL HYPERTENSION — edema, hyponatremia, decreased urine output.

GLOMERULONEPHRITIS — sodium and water retention, oliguria, dyspnea, pulmonary edema, uremic odor, myocardial hypertrophy.

thereby reducing plasma volume.

2. Sympatholytics diminish the sympathetic reflexes that produce a stepped-up heart rate and blood pressure.

3. Vasodilators relax the arterial smooth-muscle walls.

The drug chosen in each case depends on what's causing the patient's hypertension. Although antihypertensive drugs are usually used in combination, they are usually begun singly. If the patient's diastolic pressure is consistently above 90, treatment almost always begins with a diuretic. If, after a trial period of 1 to 2 months, more control is needed, the next therapeutic step would include reserpine (Serpasil) or methyldopa (Aldomet).

If the second drug added to the diuretic doesn't adequately reduce blood pressure, a third drug will be added — most likely hydralazine (Apresoline). If a patient's hypertension is traceable to a high renin secretion, then a receptor antagonist — propranolol (Inderal) — may be used instead of a diuretic from the outset. Recently, propranolol has also proven to be an effective antihypertensive agent when combined with a diuretic.

New agents for long-term management of hypertension have helped minimize disturbing side effects. Clonidine hydrochloride (Catapres), an adrenergic inhibitor, acts on the cardiorespiratory center in the brain's medulla. By stimulating alpha-adrenergic receptor sites centrally, it inhibits sympathetic outflow. Peripheral effects of this drug are diminished vasoconstriction and decreased peripheral vascular resistance. Prazosin (Minipres) relaxes peripheral arterioles and decreases total peripheral vascular resistance. The search continues for the "ideal" agent. Good control of elevated blood pressure is indispensable in forestalling cumulative target-organ damage and avoiding hypertensive crisis (see page 71).

Patient education crucial

Your hypertensive patient needs painstaking education if he's to avoid a worsening illness and repeated hospital admissions. Only if he understands his disease can he accept and respond with purpose to a treatment plan that seems superfluous to a patient without distressing symptoms.

So, always explain the pathology of hypertension and its ramifications. You've got to convince the patient that he has a lifelong illness that needs controlling, *even if he doesn't feel bad*. Ideally, include a family member when you are planning and explaining treatment. This will gain the patient greater understanding and support at home.

Then, find out how well the patient himself understands his disease, and what makes it worse. Discuss general principles of healthful living — weight control, diet, daily habits, minimizing stress. Does he understand that sodium restriction reduces blood volume and lightens the work of the heart? Does he know that caffeine is a powerful vasoconstrictor and increases the work of the heart? Does he know that coffee, tea, and cola drinks (and some ordinary medications such as Anacin tablets) all contain caffeine? Does he know that nicotine acts much like caffeine? Make sure he knows these reasons why he'll be told to give up certain things.

Patients with hypertension also need to avoid what stress they can, or learn to handle it differently. Various techniques for mitigating stress have been successful: prayer, psychotherapy, yoga, and biofeedback among them.

What about side effects?

If the patient knows what to expect, you can save him a lot of worry. For example, warn men that failure to ejaculate is commonplace with guanethidine (Ismelin) and other agents that decrease sympathetic outflow. (See Appendices for common antihypertensive drugs, their dosages, and common side effects.)

One of the most troublesome, even dangerous, effects is excessive potassium loss from diuretic therapy. This can be intensified by combining diuretics with other drugs such as corticosteroids. The first sign of it may be calf pain or leg cramps. Or the patient may complain of weakness and fatigue. To keep track of it, the doctor will order occasional checks of the patient's serum potassium level. If he doesn't order a potassium supplement, recommend foods high in potassium: orange juice, bananas, apricots, figs, raisins, meat, leafy green vegetables, and seafood. If salt is restricted but not forbidden, you may suggest Lite-Salt, a combination of sodium and potassium chloride.

In patients taking high doses of thiazide or furosemide (Lasix), serum uric acid is commonly elevated. Explain this to any patient with joint problems. Gouty symptoms can easily

Diagnostic profile
Blood pressure consistently above 140/90
Anginal pain
Edema of the extremities
Dyspnea on exertion
Retinal hemorrhages and exudates
Severe occipital headaches with nausea and vomiting, drowsiness, anxiety, and mental impairment
Late signs of associated arteriolar nephrosclerosis: polyuria, nocturia, protein and red blood cells in urine

Questions hypertensive patients ask

I like to cook with a lot of salt. How can salt harm me?
Salt (sodium) causes the body to retain water. Studies show that too much sodium and water retention increase your blood pressure, and therefore, the work of the heart.

Do I have to stop using salt entirely?
No. The body needs some sodium for normal body metabolism. We suggest a modification of salt intake: Don't add salt to your food since a surprising number of foods already contain salt. Stay away from the foods or beverages high in sodium listed on page 89.

The doctor said my blood pressure is normal now. Must I keep taking my medication? I feel so good.
The medication you're taking to lower your blood pressure has reached what we call a therapeutic level, keeping your blood pressure normal. So yes, you must keep taking your medication. If you skip doses or stop altogether, your blood pressure will rise, perhaps rapidly, requiring hospitalization.

be controlled with allopurinol (Zyloprim).

You can help with the medication schedule. The patient's doctor sets the medication schedule, but there may be much you can do to make it more acceptable or easily followed. For example, suppose the prescription says twice a day. What does twice a day mean? First thing in the morning and last thing at night, even if he gets up at 6 and goes to bed at 2? How to space the doses better and still be sure of remembering his medication? Let him offer you some suggestions. *If it's his idea, he'll be more likely to follow it.*

While you're trying to impress your patient with the need for sticking to his program and coming back for regular review, be sure to cover his whole treatment program thoroughly. Explain each of his medications and their purpose.

Home blood pressure measurement? Measuring blood pressure at home could doubtless turn some patients into "blood pressure freaks." But not many. More numerous, probably, will be the ones who don't bother to do it at all after a while. For the patients who will use it meaningfully, home blood pressure measurement can be a great help in guiding therapy. Usually, they can get truer readings when relaxed at home than when tense about the possible results in the nurse's or doctor's office. You have to use your judgment about which patients to enlist in a home measurement program. Or, select a member of the family to do the job. And emphasize that it isn't the single reading that counts, but the trend.

Nurses and community screening
The American Heart Association says that more than 7 million people in the U.S. and Canada have hypertension and don't know it. Such people may turn up at hypertensive clinics — local screening programs. Many of these clinics are managed by nurses.

We nurses can help hypertensive patients in two ways. First, by finding them. Then, by persuading them to cooperate with treatment. If we can do these well, we can change the present day statistics of poor control for excellent ones.

Coronary Artery Disease
Stages of progression

BY CHRISTINE W. CANNON, RN, MSN

WE'RE QUITE USED TO TREATING the end stage of coronary artery disease — myocardial infarction — vigorously and effectively. With the latest techniques, we can terminate ventricular fibrillation and even resuscitate after cardiac arrest. But we don't do nearly as much for patients in earlier stages of coronary artery disease. Do we ignore these earlier stages simply because they generally produce no symptoms? Or because doing something meaningful about them is much more difficult? In either case, we're not doing as much as we can.

We can do more

The most important thing we can do is help patients prevent the onset of coronary artery disease. And that's quite a challenge. The ultimate cause of coronary artery disease is still unknown, and the meaning of and methods for controlling risk factors (such as cholesterol) keep changing with ongoing scientific study. Moreover, many of the risk factors (smoking, eating habits, personality factors) are quite difficult to change, even with others' strong support. You can't guarantee that the patient will escape further illness even if he does *everything* you suggest. Despite all this, we've got to routinely

Controllable factors in C.A.D.

Hypertension greatly predisposes to coronary artery disease. As diastolic blood pressure exceeds 90 mm Hg and the systolic exceeds 140 mm Hg, the risk of coronary artery disease increases sharply. In uncontrolled hypertension, the heart must work harder to force blood from the left ventricle into the constricted peripheral circuit. Consequently, the myocardium hypertrophies, needing much more oxygen to energize the greater muscle mass of the left ventricle. Controlling blood pressure requires control of obesity, restricted salt intake, and the careful use of diuretics and antihypertensives. Uncontrolled hypertension commonly results from late diagnosis or poor compliance with recommended treatment.

Diabetes is another source of circulatory damage. Controlling it through diet and insulin aims to reduce connective tissue degeneration, which may accelerate atherogenesis; and to regulate body insulin, which may affect lipid metabolism and arterial response.

Diet may affect one risk factor, hyperlipidemia. High levels of cholesterol, triglyceride, and saturated fatty acids have been linked with increased coronary artery disease. We can recommend moderation in daily fat intake (using more polyunsaturated fats than saturated) and control of obesity. Probably the best answer is to encourage regular, vigorous physical activity to use up those ingested fats.

Smoking overstimulates the heart, constricts peripheral blood vessels, and releases carbon monoxide which interferes with myocardial oxygenation.

teach patients with coronary artery disease (CAD):
- what we know about the process of atherosclerosis
- what risk factors are and how to control them
- how to recognize, relieve, and prevent anginal attacks.

Group teaching ideal

Teaching such patients in groups helps them learn that other people share the same problems. Group discussions encourage free expression of some of the anxiety, depression, and denial common in such patients. In groups, patients can swap ideas and methods for making difficult adjustments (like tips for reducing stress and stopping smoking) — a real plus for patients struggling to control their disease by changing their life-style.

What information should *you* provide? Begin with a simple explanation of the structure and function of the heart (with emphasis on the coronary arteries). Be sure to include signs and symptoms of coronary artery disease; risk factors and how to control them; diet management; coping with stress; therapeutic exercise; and control of smoking habits. Offer helpful pamphlets such as those from the American Heart Association. You may want to make personal visits or phone calls to persons who have special problems or need special instructions.

Risk factors: Some controllable — some not

You're surely familiar with the relationship between certain "risk factors" and coronary artery disease. Risk factors are usually classified as uncontrollable (age, sex, race, and heredity) and controllable (diabetes, hypertension, hyperlipidemia, sedentary lifestyle, smoking, and stress). When teaching patients about risk factors, it's best to emphasize the controllable ones. This offers the patient hope that he *can* feel better, and something he can do to make it happen. But resist the temptation to overstate the amount of control that's attainable. For example, diet has been proclaimed the answer to one risk factor, hyperlipidemia, and low-fat, low-cholesterol diets have become popular even though some question the link between dietary habits and serum cholesterol levels. Actually, a strict low-fat diet decreases serum cholesterol by less than 10% of its baseline level, because the body synthesizes its own cholesterol. New evidence suggests that high cholesterol levels may

Map of the coronaries

The left coronary artery (LCA) arises from a single ostium. The uppermost part, which supplies the whole left side of the heart, is called the left main coronary. It bifurcates almost immediately into the left anterior descending artery (LAD) and the left circumflex artery (LCF). The LAD supplies the entire anterior surface of the left ventricle; the medial portion of the right ventricle anteriorly; the lower third of the posterior right ventricle; and the upper two-thirds of the intraventricular septum. The left circumflex supplies the lateral wall and the lower half of the posterior left ventricle; and most of the left atrium.

The right coronary artery (RCA) supplies the upper half of the posterior wall of the left ventricle and the upper portion of the right ventricle.

Left circumflex coronary artery

Left main coronary artery

Right coronary artery

Left anterior descending coronary artery

Hard-hearted
Atherosclerosis causes ninety
percent of all coronary heart
disease cases. The remaining
cases can be caused by
congenital abnormalities of the
arteries, luetic changes following
syphilitic infection, vascular
changes due to autoimmune
disorders, and coronary
embolism.

Coronary artery disease
develops through three progressive stages. 1) As early as
childhood, fatty streaks appear
in the arteries — thin, smooth,
slightly elevated yellow dots or
lines which, in some cases,
regress completely. 2) Fibrous
plaques develop, reflecting both
a low-grade inflammatory
reaction and a healing response.
This stage usually indicates that
the disease will progress further.
3) Complications develop:
necrosis, calcification, and
vascularization with or without
hemorrhage into the plaque.
Changes like these predispose
the patient to thrombosis.

actually result from impaired conversion of cholesterol into
bile acid. This conversion may be affected by certain noxious
chemicals (such as carbon monoxide) prevalent in indus-
trialized countries.

What can we reasonably recommend to patients with hyperlipidemia? We can recommend moderation in daily fat intake
(using more polyunsaturated fats); control of obesity (obesity
increases body synthesis of cholesterol); and regular, vigorous
physical activity to use up the ingested fats. Regular exercise
offers many proven benefits: reduction in heart rate, systolic
blood pressure, blood lipids, and body weight; and increases
in exercise tolerance, cardiac efficiency, fibrinolytic activity,
and overall well-being. But don't *promise* the patient that if he
exercises regularly all will be well. It may not. There's always
one patient in the cardiac rehabilitation class who announces
that he had a myocardial infarction even though he watched
his diet and jogged regularly for the last 10 years.

What can you tell patients about stress? No one can total-
ly avoid it. But patients can learn to reduce it by avoiding
noise and crowds; by changing stressful jobs; by learning to
accept what cannot be changed; by exercising to release tension (yoga, walking, or just deep-breathing exercises); by getting adequate sleep and rest; and by developing an enjoyable
hobby.

Know the uncontrollable factors

Coronary artery disease is more prevalent in whites than in
blacks; in men than in women; in middle-aged and older than in
young people (although fatty streaks in the intimal arterial
layer, the precursors of occluding plaques, can be found in the
young). Women seem to escape coronary artery disease until
after menopause, probably because of a retarding influence of
estrogen on atherogenesis. But, coronary heart disease does
seem to be rising among premenopausal women since more of
them are smoking and taking on the competitive, stress-
producing jobs traditionally held by men.

Familial tendency toward coronary artery disease seems a
strong risk factor. Many young coronary patients had fathers,
brothers, or grandfathers with premature coronary disease.
No one can change his age, race, or hereditary disposition.
But, knowing their potential effects may motivate the high-risk
candidate to control the factors he *can* change.

Recognize the coronary-prone patient

Let's consider Mr. Stern, a 48-year-old accountant. His father and brother both had died prematurely of coronary disease. But Mr. Stern liked to boast that he'd never been sick a day in his life. He loved the challenges of tax time — the phone calls, the appointments, the deadlines and, most of all, the competition with the younger accountants in his office. He smoked 3 packs of cigarettes a day to "help him relax," and boasted that he could eat almost anything — and usually did. He was 40 pounds overweight. Recently, he'd been having frequent sudden, short attacks of pressure-like "indigestion." He noticed this often while rushing back to his office after lunch, sometimes while working at his desk, and sometimes during sexual intercourse.

You won't be surprised to know that his "indigestion" was actually angina pectoris, his first warning that coronary artery disease was gradually cutting off the blood supply to his heart muscle. During cardiac evaluation studies, Mr. Stern was given a submaximal exercise stress test. He developed his typical "indigestion" after 3 minutes on the treadmill. At the same time, he developed S-T segment depression of 2 mm and S-T straightening (a positive stress test for CAD). His resting EKG appeared normal, but his resting blood pressure was 150/98. His serum cholesterol was high at 300 mg %.

What is angina?

Angina is the discomfort caused by inadequate delivery of oxygen to the myocardium (myocardial ischemia). The resulting accumulation of acid metabolites stimulates myocardial nerve endings to transmit pain to the cardiac nerves and upper thoracic posterior roots (which explains why patients can feel cardiac pain in the left shoulder and arm). Typically, the patient describes anginal pain as a sudden and transient discomfort in the anterior chest. It's brought on by exertion and relieved by rest.

Angina is not always easy to diagnose because of the varying character of the pain. But if you ask the right questions, you should be able to identify probable anginal pain. Your questions should always include these:
- Where is the pain? Point to it.
- Describe the pain: What does it feel like?
- How did it start? What brings it on? What relieves it?

Change of heart
In this cardiac cath, you can see an occlusion of the left anterior descending artery which prevented distal filling until a graft was inserted to bypass the occlusion. Grafts like this are formed by taking a vein segment (usually part of the saphenous), inverting it, and anastomosing it above and below the occlusion.

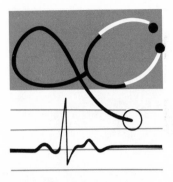

Diagnostic profile for angina
EKG abnormalities during and
after exercise
• Chest X-rays
• Cardiac catheterization
before surgery
• Nitroglycerin will shorten an
attack of anginal pain or increase
the tolerance to exercise.

STABLE ANGINA: occurs over a
long time in same pattern of onset,
duration, and intensity of
symptoms.

UNSTABLE ANGINA: frequency,
intensity, and duration of
symptoms increase as
atherosclerotic process
progresses. About 50% of
patients will infarct within 3 to 18
months after onset.

PRINZMETAL'S ANGINA: chest
discomfort at rest due to coronary
artery spasm causes transient S-T
segment elevation and pain.

ANGINA DECUBITUS: chest
discomfort that occurs in the
recumbent position, relieved by
sitting or standing.

NOCTURNAL ANGINA: occurs only
at night, but not necessarily in the
recumbent position.

INTRACTABLE ANGINA: chronic
chest discomfort that is physically
incapacitating, and refractory to
medical treatment.

• Does the pain seem to move? Where?

• Have you had the same pain before? How long did it last?

• Do you have any other symptoms or discomfort? (Look for signs of shortness of breath, profuse sweating, and nausea.)

Classically, anginal pain occurs substernally with radiation down the left arm and lasts 3 to 5 minutes. Patients describe it as heavy, squeezing, constricting, choking, smothering, expanding, aching, or burning; some simply say "something's not right in my chest." Some patients just can't seem to find the right words, so watch for nonverbal clues as well. A grimace with a fist clenched against the sternum is one reliable nonverbal clue. You can almost count on angina pectoris when you see it.

Anginal pain usually occurs during exertion, emotional stress, isometric exercises, and stressful dream states. It's especially likely when the patient is cold or digesting a meal. Other factors which can bring on an anginal attack include anger, fright, and strong emotion — all of which increase myocardial oxygen consumption. Remember that oxygen needs are chronically exaggerated in aortic-valve disease accompanied by left ventricular hypertrophy, obesity, hypertension, anemia, hyperthyroidism, and hypoxemia from chronic lung disease. Anginal pain may radiate to the neck, jaw, shoulder, elbow, down the arm — especially the left — or even to the fingers. Remember that patients with angina pectoris need not describe their pain in classic terms and they can feel such pain anywhere between the jaw and epigastrium.

Chest pain: Anginal or not?

Chest pain may signal a variety of disorders, but your first concern is always to decide whether or not the pain is anginal. Always ask the patient:

• *Is the pain better or worse when you breathe in or out?* Anginal pain isn't.

• *Is the pain better or worse when you change your body position?* Again, anginal pain usually isn't.

The pain of angina and myocardial infarction is unaffected by changes in position. But pain of pericarditis decreases when the patient sits or leans forward; it increases when he lies on his left side, laughs, or coughs.

• *Does the pain seem deep or superficial; mild or intense?*

Cardiac pain seems deep and unusually intense; noncardiac pain is typically described as mild "soreness" or dull aching.

• *Can you point to the pain with one finger?* Cardiac pain tends to be diffuse, not sharply localized.

If you're present during an actual anginal attack, your assessment should include physical signs, vital signs, and an EKG. The patient may look normal, but more likely obviously distressed. Generally, he looks quite pale and has cool, perspiring skin. His pulse and blood pressure may be elevated, especially if the angina comes on after exertion. In some patients examined during an actual attack of angina, you may hear an atrial gallop (S_4). In some patients, you can detect these vibrations only when the patient is in the left lateral position. Some patients have ventricular gallop (S_3), suggesting a temporary decompensation of the left ventricle. In some, the S_3 and S_4 sounds may merge to form a summation gallop.

Your responsibility to a patient with angina includes prompt action to relieve pain. Help the patient into a comfortable resting position (with his head elevated) and give oxygen. The patient with confirmed angina needs a sublingual nitroglycerin tablet at the first hint of pain, and another one at 5 minute intervals if pain persists. Be supportive and offer realistic reassurance. Be sympathetic. But don't tell the patient that everything will be alright, when everything clearly is not. Above all, stay with him until the attack subsides.

Between attacks, the patient should keep a few nitroglycerin tablets with him at all times and at his bedside (in a tightly closed, dark glass bottle). He can then take them as needed to relieve or prevent angina. Warn the patient that nitroglycerin may cause reflex tachycardia, a pounding headache, flushing, and occasional dizziness. And warn against standing for about 30 minutes after taking it (and standing up *suddenly* thereafter) because it may cause postural hypotension.

Of course, preventing an attack is always better than dealing with one after it happens. So you must help patients identify those activities that trigger angina. For Mr. Stern, trigger activities included any exercise (walking, sexual intercourse) soon after meals and stress, usually accompanied by cigarette smoking. He was encouraged to relax — whenever he felt the demands of his work were "getting to him," to go outside and deeply breathe some fresh air for 5 or 10 minutes. He was

HDL: New heart-risk key

A new lab test predictive of coronary heart disease measures serum high density lipoproteins (HDL) in conjunction with serum cholesterol levels. HDL, it appears, inhibits the entry of cholesterol into arterial cells. It also increases the rate at which cholesterol leaves the cells.

A ratio of 5 total cholesterol to HDL reflects a "standard" risk; of 10 doubles the risk; and of 20 triples the risk, with a likelihood of triple-vessel coronary disease. A desirable ratio is 3.5 or less.

When considered alone, an HDL level of 45 mg% in men and 55 mg% in women is standard. (The higher HDL levels in women may reflect their lesser predisposition to coronary disease.) Preventive care now involves raising HDL levels (largely through exercise) as much as lowering total serum cholesterol.

Haste makes waste

Cardiologists have identified a personality type that's especially vulnerable to acute myocardial infarctions. They call it a Type A personality. A Type A person has "hurry-up sickness," a malignant compulsion to achieve as much as possible in as little time as possible.

Interestingly, a Type A person has an increased secretion of catecholamines such as norepinephrine and vanillylmandelic acid (VMA), high fasting levels of triglycerides, betalipoproteins, and cholesterol, and a slow clearance of fat from the blood. His blood even clots faster than normal. But when a Type A person modifies his behavior patterns, all these findings reverse themselves.

You can identify a Type A personality by the following traits: He is chronically impatient — he talks, walks, and eats quickly; his mind is always active; he can converse only on topics that interest him; he is fiercely competitive; he feels guilty for relaxing. A Type A person will perform many activities at once to save time — like watching TV as he reads the newspaper during a meal. If you notice such behavior in your patient, bring it to his attention and try to help him modify his lifestyle.

advised he could prevent angina during intercourse by getting into better physical condition with regular, prescribed exercise and by using nitroglycerin just before. To reduce his baseline myocardial oxygen requirements, Mr. Stern needed to reduce his weight and blood pressure, and stop smoking.

Mr. Stern's drug regimen included vasodilation with short- and long-acting nitrates, isosorbide dinitrate (Isordil), 5 mg sublingually, one hour after meals and at bedtime. He was to supplement sublingual Isordil with the routine application of 1" of nitroglycerin paste applied to his chest wall every 6 hours. He could augment these long-acting nitrates with sublingual nitroglycerin for rapid onset. Sublingual nitroglycerin has a short duration of action, so it may need to be repeated once or twice every 5 minutes during an anginal attack. Mr. Stern also took propranolol (Inderal), 20 mg four times a day, 30 minutes before meals and at bedtime to reduce myocardial oxygen demands by decreasing heart rate and contractility and blood pressure. Taken before meals (food interferes with absorption), its onset (45 minutes) and duration of action (5 hours) coincided with Mr. Stern's most active times and with the onset of Isordil. Incidentally, when Inderal and Isordil are used together, they cancel out each other's adverse effects: Isordil's vasodilating effect opposed Inderal's tendency to reduce myocardial blood flow; Inderal prevents Isordil's reflex, oxygen-consuming tachycardia.

He also began an exercise program that included 3 sessions a week of monitored exercise vigorous enough to increase heart rate, but not to cause angina. Unfortunately, he began to have longer, more frequent, and more easily triggered anginal episodes. During one of these sessions, he developed a full-blown anginal attack (with S-T segment depression, S_3 gallop rhythm, rales at both lung bases, and BP, 190/105). He was then hospitalized for unstable (pre-infarction) angina. Because half of the patients with such angina develop an infarct within 18 months of onset, cardiac catheterization was ordered to evaluate coronary bypass surgery. It showed extensive narrowing of the right coronary artery and an ominous lesion in the proximal left coronary artery (left main-stem lesion). Fortunately, the left circumflex and anterior descending vessels were patent; his bypass operation was a success. Even so, Mr. Stern had to learn to live within strict limits to control risk factors and prevent the return of angina.

Acute Myocardial Infarction
Severe ASHD

BY CATHERINE CIAVERELLI MANZI, RN

YOU'VE JUST TAKEN A CALL from the rescue squad. They're on their way with a middle-aged man who collapsed on the street. Their tentative diagnosis: acute myocardial infarction. Do you feel competent to cope? Do you know what physical changes to expect? What symptoms to look for and what they mean? What lab data will be pertinent and how to interpret the results? What complications are possible and how to guard against them? And, of course, what treatment is likely to be used so you can be ready to give it promptly?

If you can confidently answer yes to all these questions, the care you give patients with acute myocardial infarction (AMI) is quite probably lifesaving. But if you can't, you may find this review helpful.

Chest pain typical

Patients with an AMI usually have severe chest pain. This pain differs from that of angina pectoris in that it lasts longer than 20 minutes. Most angina subsides in only a few minutes. The pain of AMI usually persists from one-half hour to several hours; rarely, it may last no longer than 5 minutes. Such pain or discomfort may begin anytime, during effort, rest, or sleep.

What happens in acute MI

As you know, when atherosclerosis narrows or obstructs the coronary arteries, blood flow to the myocardium — and oxygen along with it — decreases. Ischemia and then necrosis develop in that portion of the myocardium that's not adequately nourished. This is an acute myocardial infarction.

An AMI jeopardizes the heart's pumping mechanism. What you'll find hemodynamically includes a decrease in arterial pressure, stroke volume, ejection fraction of the myocardium, and cardiac output.

Of course, pressure in the ventricles during diastole is called preload or left ventricular filling pressure. Afterload refers to systemic blood pressure and systemic vascular resistance. To pump effectively, the left ventricle must overcome this resistance. But since myocardial damage compromises contractility, both preload and afterload increase along with end-diastolic and end-systolic volumes.

Although an MI may not disturb ventricular function in some patients, life-threatening alterations in function can occur abruptly. So even though your patient may have a normal blood pressure, make sure you monitor him closely during this critical period.

The pain of AMI is generally substernal but may occur anywhere in the anterior chest, back, epigastrium, jaw, neck, elbow, shoulder, wrist, or forearm. The patient may describe his discomfort as a feeling of heaviness, burning, aching, choking, constriction, tightness, crushing, squeezing, or expanding. He is likely to use expressions such as, "like someone sitting on my chest," "a tight rubber band around my chest," or "feeling as if my arm would break." He may also report weakness or numbness in one or both arms.

Although severe chest pain is classically typical of myocardial infarction, roughly 15% of patients with AMI present with atypical pain or virtually no symptoms at all. I remember Mr. Bradford who was admitted to the CCU to rule out a diagnosis of AMI. He denied having any chest pain or arm pain. But when his nurse asked, "Is anything bothering you?" he said, "Yes, my jaw aches." His jaw pain, in fact, represented ischemic pain; serial electrocardiograms confirmed an acute myocardial infarction.

Other atypical symptoms of MI can include syncope, vertigo, nausea, vomiting, dyspnea, diaphoresis, pallor, hypotension, and hypertension. Fever is extremely rare at the onset of myocardial infarction but does sometimes occur in the first few days after the infarct. Remember, such fever rarely exceeds 101° F. (38.3° C.). A higher temperature (102° F., 33.3° C.) or persistent rise suggests complications. Notify the doctor and consider other causes.

Changes in heart sounds typical

Some patients at the onset of an AMI look normal and have normal blood pressure, pulse, and heart sounds. More usually, however, cardiac auscultation reveals characteristic changes: alterations in the intensity of heart sounds; atrial gallop (S_4); ventricular gallop (S_3); and, an apical systolic murmur (indicating papillary muscle dysfunction of one or both ventricles).

Patients with AMI may or may not have symptoms related to mitral regurgitation (primarily those associated with left ventricular failure and pulmonary congestion: dyspnea, rales, edema). This murmur is heard best over the mitral valve area (left side of the chest wall between the 5th and 6th intercostal space). It may be localized to the apex or transmitted to the left of the sternal border or to the axilla. It has a high-pitched or blowing quality but does not have to be holosystolic (persisting

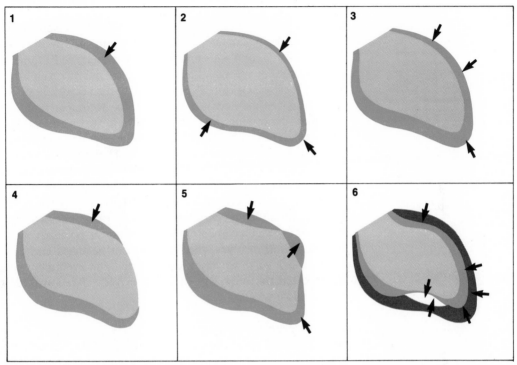

throughout systole) as is the rheumatic mitral regurgitant murmur.

The doctor will locate precordial and systolic movement of the ventricle by percussing and palpating the apex, the left and right sternal borders, the suprasternal notch, and the subxiphoid. He will look for the precordial bulge that can accompany an AMI. This bulge is due to the paradoxical motion of the infarcted myocardium.

After physical examination, patients suspected of having had a myocardial infarction always need confirming diagnostic studies. Such studies include enzyme analysis and serial EKGs. Enzyme analysis aims to detect characteristic changes in tissue levels of SGOT, LDH, and CPK (see page 88).

EKG pattern diagnostic

Q waves representing normal septal depolarization are considered normal, when seen in the left precordial leads and leads aVL, L1. When the Q wave is wider than 0.04 seconds (one small block on the graph paper) or deeper than 1 mm (1 small

The ins and outs
1. A *normal heart* contracts in a strong uniform motion. But a heart damaged by an MI can develop left ventricular dysynergy or asynergy. 2. A *hypokinetic* contraction remains uniform but lacks force. 3. *Asyneresis* refers to a localized hypokinetic contraction. 4. *Akinesis* is the failure of a portion of the ventricular wall to contract. 5. *Dyskinesis* means a paradoxical systolic expansion or bulging of part of the ventricular wall.
6. *Asynchrony* refers to the disturbed temporal sequence of contraction.

blocks), it's considered abnormal and diagnostic for myocardial necrosis. Whenever you see abnormal waves on an EKG, record their appearance, depth, and width, and notify the doctor. Watch for a wide and deep Q wave with S-T segment elevation or T wave inversion — the typical infarction pattern. Expect these changes in leads oriented to the necrotic area. In leads opposite the necrotic area, look for accompanying S-T segment depression and an upright T wave (reciprocal changes). These changes represent the indirect current of injury. Look for reciprocal changes first. They're usually more obvious and will alert you to look for S-T elevation — often a more subtle change.

Infarcts can occur in the anterior, lateral, posterior, or inferior walls of the myocardium either singly or in combination (anterior-lateral location is common). When an acute myocardial infarction resolves, the S-T segment becomes less elevated; the T wave becomes less inverted and eventually upright. Often the only EKG sign of an old infarction is the pathologic q wave.

Life-threatening complications
Anticipate and watch for complications carefully, since early diagnosis and proper management may decide whether or not the patient survives.

● *Ventricular arrhythmia* is the most common and the most perilous complication. Watch for PVCs (premature ventricular contractions) that may precede ventricular tachycardia. They need immediate treatment. Ventricular arrhythmias may follow myocardial ischemia, hypotension, impaired pulmonary ventilation, or drug therapy. When ventricular tachycardia is the first sign of an AMI, it forecasts a tendency to shock and congestive heart failure.

● *Other arrhythmias* can also complicate AMI: atrial tachycardia, atrial flutter or fibrillation, varying degrees of A-V heart block, and sinus bradycardia. These arrhythmias usually relate to the site of the infarction and the involved arteries. For example, atrial infarction involving the right coronary artery proximal to the sinus node artery usually fosters atrial arrhythmias. Inferior infarctions usually foster A-V block. Left anterior hemi-block, and right bundle-branch block may result from anterior infarction.

● *Heart failure* (mild dysfunction of the left ventricle [LVD]).

Infarctions in different sites of the heart cause EKG changes. Recognizing these changes will help you assess your patient.

- An *inferior wall myocardial infarction* will show typical pattern changes — a pathological Q wave, S-T segment elevation, and T wave inversion — in leads II, III, and aVF.
- Sometimes an inferior or posterior wall infarction will involve the lateral wall as well. *Lateral wall involvement* will cause a reduced R wave, a T wave inversion, and, in some cases, an elevation of the S-T segment, in the lateral leads V₅, V₆, aVL, and L₁.
- A *posterior wall infarction* causes a mirror image of the normal precordial EKG pattern.

CHARACTERISTIC EKGs IN MI

- An *anterior MI* will produce a typical infarction pattern in leads I, aVL, and V₂ to V₆.
- An *anterior septal infarction* will cause the typical pattern in leads V₂ to V₄.
- An *anterior lateral infarction* will produce the typical pattern in leads I, V₅, and V₆.
- An infarction within the anterior lateral surface of the left ventricle — *a high anterolateral infarction* — will produce typical changes in leads aVL, L₁, and V₆.

Change for the better
These EKG patterns gradually return to normal. Recovery after an MI can be divided into four phases:

PHASE I (the acute phase): Immediately after onset or within 48 hours, leads oriented to the injured area show abnormal Q waves, an elevated S-T segment, and inverted T waves. Reciprocal changes, such as S-T depression, occur in leads oriented to the uninjured area.

PHASE II: This phase covers the gradual return of the elevated S-T segment to the baseline.

PHASE III: All T waves return to normal or near-normal configuration.

PHASE IV (the stabilized phase): Here an abnormal Q wave may be the only sign of an infarction.

These four phases may be complete in 3 days or may take as long as 10. Remember always to interpret EKGs in light of other laboratory findings and the patient's symptoms.

COMMON ARRHYTHMIAS

PACs

Treatment: Often none, but quinidine may be used

AV BLOCK — SECOND DEGREE

Treatment: Atropine, Isuprel, or pacemaker

PVCs

Treatment: Lidocaine or atropine

PAT

Treatment: Carotid sinus pressure, propranolol, or metaraminol

AV BLOCK — THIRD DEGREE

Treatment: Atropine, Isuprel, or pacemaker

VENTRICULAR TACHYCARDIA

Treatment: Cardioversion (except for patients on digitalis) or lidocaine

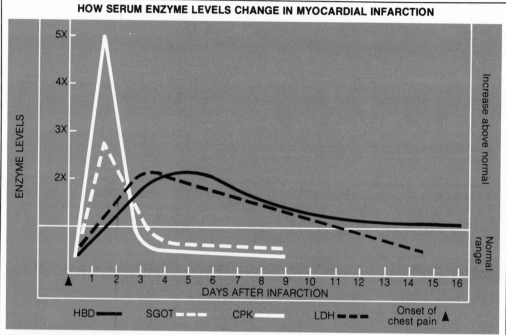

HOW SERUM ENZYME LEVELS CHANGE IN MYOCARDIAL INFARCTION

Increase above normal

Normal range

ENZYME LEVELS

5X
4X
3X
2X

1 2 3 4 5 6 7 8 9 10 11 12 13 14 15 16
DAYS AFTER INFARCTION

HBD —— SGOT ---- CPK —— LDH ■■■■ Onset of chest pain ▲

Cardiac enzymes: critical clues
Patients suspected of having a myocardial infarction always need serial EKGs and serial enzyme studies. Enzymes are catalytic proteins that vary in concentration, depending upon the tissue in which they appear. Since a damaged tissue releases enzymes into the blood, enzyme studies tell what organ is damaged and to what extent.

Draw blood samples for an enzyme study very carefully, since a traumatic venipuncture can falsely elevate results. For example, red blood cells which contain LDH, HBD, and SGOT, can release these enzymes in cases of hemolysis.

Look for three highly specific enzymes to help diagnose a myocardial infarction:
SGOT — serum glutamic-oxaloacetic transaminase, an enzyme found mainly in the heart muscle and the liver and to some degree in skeletal muscle, kidney, and red blood cells. Normal value: 8 to 40u/ml (Karmen unit); 6 to 18 I.U./L.

LDH — lactic dehydrogenase, found in the heart, liver, kidney, brain, skeletal muscle, and erythrocytes. Since it's found in tissues outside the heart, laboratories separate LDH into five subgroups called isoenzymes. The LDH_1 and LDH_2 isoenzymes are the myocardial fraction that rises after myocardial infarction. Some laboratories routinely measure hydroxy-butyrate dehydrogenase (HBD) as an indirect measure of LDH_1 and LDH_2. Normal value: 150 to 450u/ml (Wroblewski unit); 71 to 207 I.U./L.; 80 to 120 (Wacker units).

CPK — creatine phosphokinase occurs in the heart, skeletal muscle, and brain, but not in red blood cells or the liver. CPK levels rise after hard exercise, polymyositis, muscular dystrophy, muscle injury, and myocardial infarction. After skeletal muscle abnormalities and cerebral disease are ruled out, *elevated CPK is considered specific for myocardial damage.* However, remember, intramuscular injections *alone* can elevate the CPK enzyme level. So avoid such injections in patients being studied for possible acute myocardial infarction. For this reason, some hospitals routinely give such patients analgesic medication intravenously. Some laboratories solve this problem by separating CPK into skeletal (CPK-MM) or cardiac muscle (CPK-MB) fractions.
Normal value: Male, 0 to 50 milliunits/ml (I.U. at 30° C.); female, 0 to 30 milliunits/ml (I.U. at 30° C.); CPK-MB = 15% of total; CPK-MM = 85% of total.

Watch for its signs: atrial (S₄) or ventricular (S₃) gallop rhythm, neck-vein distention, pulsus alternans, and pulmonary rales. Mortality rate is 80% in patients with an AMI who develop congestive failure and pump failure (cardiogenic shock).

• *Pulmonary edema* (moderate LVD) follows left-sided heart failure. When the left side of the heart can't maintain adequate venous output, the result is increased pulmonary artery pressure and pulmonary congestion. Its physical signs include dyspnea, bibasilar pulmonary rales, oliguria, and tachycardia.

• *Pump failure* (severe LVD) occurs when myocardial infarction damages the heart's ability to pump blood into the aorta in sufficient volume and pressure. Decreased cardiac output and inadequate tissue perfusion produce cardiogenic shock (in 10 to 15% of AMI patients). Anticipate pump failure and watch for its telltale signs: hypotension, pallor, diaphoresis, cool, clammy skin, oliguria, tachycardia, and weak, thready, rapid pulse. Such patients may also appear confused or obtunded (see also Chapter 10).

• *Pulmonary embolism* may occur in patients with recurrent bouts of congestive heart failure in patients with AMI. Suspect it when

— cyanosis is present

— heart failure doesn't respond to treatment

— unexplained pleural effusion occurs

— the patient has been on prolonged bed rest.

To prevent pulmonary embolism, encourage patients to move and exercise their legs gently and wiggle their toes. They may benefit from antiembolism stockings. Tell such patients not to cross their legs. If they are too weak to move, give regular passive exercises to the legs, and turn them from side to side often.

• *Rupture of the heart* accounts for 10% of the AMI fatalities in the hospital. This fatal complication usually occurs within the first week after transmural infarction (involving the whole myocardial wall). Its signs include sudden worsening of the patient's condition, dyspnea, shock, and distended neck veins accompanied by pulsus paradoxus. Auscultation of the chest wall may reveal murmurs and thrills. Death can follow suddenly from cardiac tamponade (see Chapter 10). If you auscultate a patient with cardiac tamponade, you may find electromechanical dissociation, electrical rhythmic activity with-

Heart-saving diet

An MI patient must watch his diet. His doctor will most likely restrict his sodium intake, so have him *avoid* the following:

• salted "snack" foods such as potato chips, peanuts

• canned soups and vegetables

• dried fruits

• delicatessen foods, especially lox and ham

• prepared foods such as TV dinners

• preserved meat (such as hot dogs) and luncheon meats

• cheeses of all kinds (including cottage)

• anything preserved in brine, such as olives, pickles, and sauerkraut.

In addition, a patient watching calories should *avoid*

• sugar and sweets

• high cholesterol foods

• milk, milk products, and coconut oil

• alcohol.

His diet should *include* the following foods, low in sodium:

Fruits and their juices

apples	apricots
bananas	dates
grapefruit	nectarines
oranges	prunes
raisins	watermelon

Vegetables (fresh or frozen)

asparagus	beans
brussels sprouts	cabbage
cauliflower	corn
lima beans	peas
peppers	potatoes
radishes	squash

Treatment goals

Your goal for treating MI patients includes relieving distress and reducing cardiac work to allow healing and prevent extension of the infarct or complications. You can promote these goals by

• *Relieving pain,* usually with morphine, 2 to 4 mg dose, I.V. or I.M.: Morphine reduces anxiety, and decreases cardiac work load. It also depresses respiration, reduces myocardial contractility and, by vasodilation, decreases blood pressure and slows the heart rate.

Meperidine hydrochloride (Demerol) is often used because it produces less nausea and respiratory depression than morphine — despite its anticholinergic-like effect which may increase the ventricular rate in patients with atrial fibrillation. Avoid inducing hypoxia, which can induce ventricular fibrillation and cardiac arrest.

• *Promoting rest:* A reduced work load will help heal the damaged myocardium and develop collateral circulation. Promote cardiac rest by enforcing bedrest as needed (especially a challenge with an active patient who's suddenly immobilized).

Once pain has subsided, encourage patients to move their feet and legs to minimize the risk of thrombophlebitis. To check on readiness for graduated activity, watch for pain, tachycardia or increased blood pressure before, during, and after activity. With patients on digoxin (Lanoxin) or propranolol (Inderal), watch closely for signs such as pain, heart rhythm changes, or shortness of breath. If these result, the patient isn't ready to resume normal activity.

(continued, opposite page)

out palpable pulses or measurable blood pressure.

• *Rupture of the interventricular septum* accounts for 2% of all deaths within the first week after AMI. This is due to new or old occlusion of both anterior and posterior descending arteries that supply most of the septal myocardium with blood. Watch for rapidly developing left heart failure, dyspnea, shock, and a harsh systolic murmur at the 4th left sternal border.

• *Papillary muscle rupture* is another severe complication with rapidly developing dyspnea, pulmonary edema, mitral insufficiency, and signs of decreased cardiac output.

• *Ventricular aneurysm* usually involves the left ventricle (95% of the time). Its clinical features include: intractable failure, angina and arrhythmias (especially sinus tachycardia and PVCs), gallop rhythm, and a palpable systolic precordial bulge.

• *Pericarditis* occurs in 15% of patients with AMI. A pericardial friction rub appears 2 to 3 days postinfarction. It produces a pain over the precordium that is aggravated by inspiration and movement. Listen for a sound like sandpaper rubbing together. The patient who develops pericarditis usually thinks he's developing another infarction and becomes quite anxious. Remember to reassure him. This pain is distinguishable from angina: It's clearly related to a change in position or breathing. It worsens during inspiration and lessens as the patient sits up in bed. The patient with pericarditis usually points to the site of pain with one finger.

• *Dressler (postmyocardial infarction)* syndrome can occur weeks or months later. The patient develops pericardial pain, pericardial friction rub, fever, left pleural effusion, arthralgia, elevated sedimentation rate, and increased serum WBCs. This syndrome needs diagnosis to separate it from a recurring AMI, pulmonary infarction, or congestive heart failure. This syndrome is thought to be due to an antigen-antibody reaction to necrotic myocardium. Its symptoms may chronically recur and may require treatment with steroids.

Emotional problems prominent

Today, most people know what a myocardial infarction means and what its consequences are. Their natural response to it is fear and anxiety that endanger an already damaged heart. Stress releases catecholamines which increase the heart rate, the force of myocardial contraction, and myocardial metabolic requirements. If the diseased heart can't cope with the greater demand for oxygen, it may develop arrhythmias, angina, heart failure, pump failure, or another myocardial infarction. Clearly, patients should try to keep anxiety within tolerable limits if they're to recover.

Some patients manage their anxiety by denying their illness. Denial relieves anxiety by reducing the threat of dying, the loss of masculinity in the male patient, the loss of health, and the fear of being a burden. Denial is common in the first 24 to 48 hours but may persist into convalescence. When it lasts longer than 2 weeks, it can seriously endanger the patient's welfare.

I remember one champion disbeliever, Mr. Stern. He was admitted to the CCU with an acute anterior-wall myocardial infarction. His hospital course was initially uneventful and he seemed pleasantly jovial. Only after a few days did we notice that he'd talk about everything *except* his illness or its treatment. Whenever we tried to talk to him about those matters, Mr. Stern merely laughed and told jokes.

The dangerous thing about denial is that it lets patients ignore the doctor's instructions. Mr. Stern ignored his need for bedrest. He often got out of bed, unplugged his monitor, and walked to the bathroom. When reprimanded, he only laughed, saying, "I'm fine, just a little tired and short of breath. I need to walk around." His nurse explained that fatigue, shortness of breath, chest pain, and increased heart rate were caused by damage to his heart — not too much rest. She repeatedly emphasized the need for rest and did finally convince him to accept the reality of his illness.

Once denial subsides and reality sets in, depression is likely to follow. The patient who realizes how illness will change his life is likely to feel sad, angry, or guilty. He may say things like, "Why did this happen to me? If only I had listened…quit smoking…found another job." Remember that many patients — particularly men — will need help in expressing such feelings for fear of seeming less than brave.

Caring for a depressed patient is extremely difficult and often frustrating. Don't let your frustration lead to over-protecting or doing everything for the patient. Instead, let him know you recognize and understand his sad feelings but expect him to function as he is capable. Being forced to do things for himself eases feelings of helplessness and gradually re-

• *Preserving myocardium:* Vasodilators — nitrates (sublingual or ointment) — increase coronary blood flow and myocardial oxygen perfusion; and maintain long-term artery dilation to meet metabolic needs. Nitrates produce more venous than arterial dilation. Nipride I.V. dilates arterial vascular beds more than venous; decreases left ventricular filling pressure (preload); and decreases peripheral vascular resistance (afterload), causing increased cardiac output and decreased blood pressure.

In AMI patients without left ventricular dysfunction, beta-adrenergic blockers such as propranolol (Inderal) reduce myocardial oxygen consumption by decreasing heart rate and contractility.

If you find a 10% increase in heart rate or a systolic blood pressure under 110 mm Hg in these patients, notify the doctor immediately.

• *Combatting arrhythmias:* Lethal arrhythmias are common after AMI. Treat ventricular arrhythmias with lidocaine (Xylocaine) or procainamide (Pronestyl). Heart block may be treated with atropine or a pacemaker (temporary or permanent), depending on the kind of heart block, the site of infarction, and the patient's clinical status.

• *Restricting diet:* A liquid or soft diet, easily digestible foods, reduces cardiac work load.

• *Giving oxygen:* Oxygen may be given (6 to 8 L per minute), usually by nasal cannula or mask for respiratory insufficiency, dyspnea, angina, shock, or cyanosis.

Questions MI patients ask

Will I be able to go back to work?
Depending on the extent of heart damage and the demands of your job, you may be able to return to work; many patients do. Or you may be able to shift duties, taking on a less demanding job.

Can I continue my normal activities, such as golf, swimming, and the like?
Moderate exercise is beneficial if it doesn't cause pain, shortness of breath, unusual fatigue, or other such symptoms. Get medical clearance, start slowly, build up gradually, and continue daily. Rest when you tire.

Will I have another heart attack?
No one knows for sure. Chances of living a full, healthy life are better if you follow your doctor's instructions.

stores confidence.

A special problem in men with an acute myocardial infarction: the threat to self-image and sexual adequacy. Such anxiety may appear as aggressive sexual behavior, a compensatory reaction. Instead of focusing on inappropriate behavior, try to help the patient find other ways to feel more competent and independent. Let him participate in planning his care and diet. Resuming some responsibility for his own care may reduce the need to prove masculinity.

Your role as teacher

Throughout the patient's stay in the hospital, take primary responsibility for explaining what he can expect from the staff, what kind of information he should report, necessary procedures, monitors, and other equipment, his activity, diet, fluid restriction, and so forth. Be sure to plan, prepare, and educate the patient and his family how to live with his illness after he goes home (see Appendices).

And don't forget to explain and prepare the patient for any moves *within* the hospital. Most patients with AMI after a few days of intensive care become conscious of their dependence on the nursing staff. They become secure in the CCU. When their condition stabilizes and they are moved to another unit, they react with great anxiety, feeling abandoned. This move can be traumatic, even dangerous, unless you prepare them for it. Don't forget their relatives, who can help support and reassure at this time. Most of all, AMI patients need to know that even after the move, CCU personnel will be available to answer any questions and give any special help needed during recovery.

Congestive Failure
Severe cardiac impairment

BY LAUREN MARIE ISACSON, RN and
KLAUS J. SCHULZ, MD

CONGESTIVE HEART FAILURE (CHF) and its most devastating extreme, pulmonary edema, are among the most common cardiovascular problems. Their symptoms are always distressing and often potentially life-threatening. You should know how to deal with these symptoms promptly and, of course, to recognize congestive failure in all its stages. This chapter will tell you how.

Sometimes insidious

In its advanced stages, CHF is easy to recognize; as full-blown pulmonary edema, its textbook symptoms are almost impossible to miss. More often, though, chronic congestive heart failure has an insidious onset. Many patients with early congestive failure complain of having a slight cold they're unable to "shake." They may have a cough combined with some wheezing, and may have even been treated for a suspected allergy. But detailed questioning usually brings out more definitive symptoms: typically, ankle edema that appears in the evening and disappears by morning (so it may not show if you examine the patient early in the day); nocturia; and anorexia. Their anorexia may be secondary to engorgement of the liver which may be palpable and slightly tender. A mild blow against the right lower lateral rib cage discloses tenderness of the liver even when it's not easily palpable or markedly enlarged. At this stage, physical examination may reveal a few rales in the lungs and not much else. If such patients are weight-conscious, they usually report a puzzling, steady weight gain.

What causes these symptoms?
CHF can result from any condition that impairs cardiac function — most commonly arteriosclerotic heart disease, myocardial infarction, hypertension, rheumatic valvular disease, or congenital heart anomalies. In most patients with these diseases, the left ventricle becomes damaged and eventually fails. Blood backs up in the left atrium and the pulmonary capillary bed. The lungs act as a sponge and take up some of this extra fluid. Eventually they, too, become overloaded and symptoms of pulmonary edema begin.

Left-sided failure is the kind most likely after myocardial infarction. Its symptoms reflect: increased pulmonary congestion and pressure, and decreased blood flow to all tissues and organs. In such patients, expect to see: dyspnea on exertion or at rest, tachypnea, orthopnea, paroxysmal nocturnal dyspnea, cough, pulmonary rales, (which may be audible without a stethoscope), fatigue, mental confusion, sodium and water retention, and decreased tolerance to physical activity.

Right-sided failure often follows left-sided failure because the right side must then pump against the increased resistance in the pulmonary system. Patients with right-sided failure typically develop dependent edema, coolness of the extremities, hepatomegaly, occasional abdominal pain, ascites, neck-vein distention, and increased venous pressure. They usually show a positive hepatojugular reflux. The tell-tale sign is neck-vein distention when the patient is upright. Neck veins may show abnormal pulsations, look distended, and feel rigid — all signs of high venous pressure.

In many elderly people, who tend to have both arteriosclerosis and some degenerative changes due to age, both ventricles begin to fail at the same time. Both chambers falter in their capacity to pump blood into the circulation; consequently, symptoms of left and right ventricular failure develop simultaneously. In such patients, the symptoms may not, at first, clearly suggest CHF.

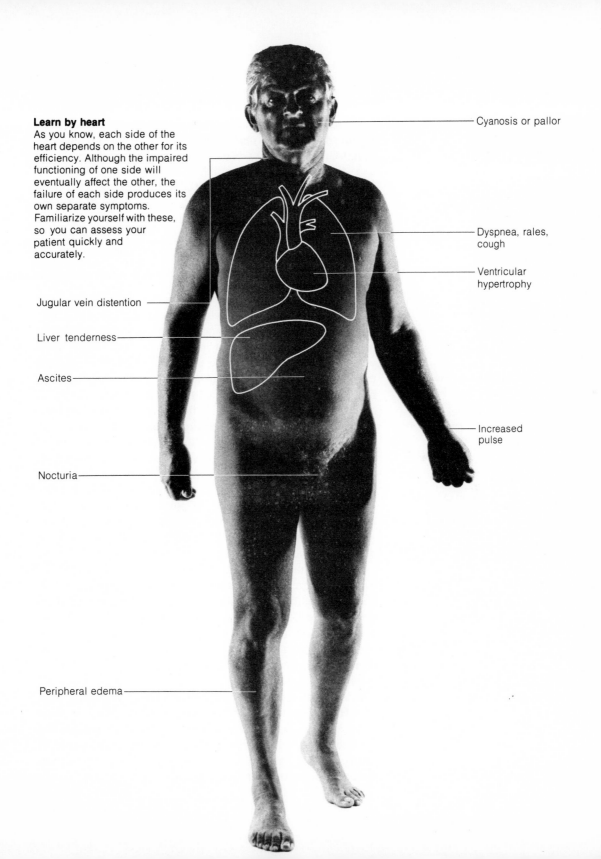

Learn by heart
As you know, each side of the heart depends on the other for its efficiency. Although the impaired functioning of one side will eventually affect the other, the failure of each side produces its own separate symptoms. Familiarize yourself with these, so you can assess your patient quickly and accurately.

Cyanosis or pallor

Dyspnea, rales, cough

Ventricular hypertrophy

Jugular vein distention

Liver tenderness

Ascites

Increased pulse

Nocturia

Peripheral edema

Pleural effusion
Roughly one-third of the patients
with congestive heart failure
develop pleural effusion — a
collection of fluid in the pleural
lining of the lungs. How does this
happen? In patients with CHF,
high venous pressure obstructs
lymphatic absorption of the fluid
that lubricates the pleura and
causes this fluid to accumulate.

You can't easily see a pleural
effusion on an X-ray unless more
than 300 ml of fluid have
accumulated; then you may see
some elevation of lung contours.
But you should be able to notice
the reduction or absence of breath
sounds at the base of the lung
where the fluid collects. If it
accumulates quickly, it may
actually shift the mediastinum to
one side, displacing the lungs
and causing dyspnea. A patient in
this situation may have an
irregular breathing pattern.

Treatment aims to correct the
congestive heart failure. Still,
good pulmonary hygiene is
important. Tell the patient to avoid
lying on the side of the effusion to
allow lung expansion and prevent
atelectasis. If he's short of breath,
he'll feel better in upright or
semi-Fowler's position. Aspiration
by thoracentesis may be needed.

Mrs. Bradford's case illustrates such insidious onset: Mrs.
Bradford was quite upset when she came to her doctor's
office. She had always been an active, healthy woman, and
had enjoyed raising her children, cooking the extravagant
meals her family loved, and successfully running a rooming
house. At age 62, she saw no reason to slow down. But for the
last 6 months, she'd been plagued by a persistent "cold." She
tired easily, was often short of breath, and from time to time
had an annoying cough, especially at night. Lately, she had to
use three pillows under her head to get any rest. She'd been
treated for "allergies," but nothing seemed to help.

Mrs. Bradford's physical examination quickly identified the
source of her problems: Auscultation and percussion revealed
left ventricular enlargement and a systolic murmur. Inspection
revealed other signs of right heart failure: a distended neck
vein, an enlarged liver, positive hepatojugular reflux, and
marked peripheral edema. Further tests confirmed congestive
heart failure: Her EKG showed a rapid heart rate (120 BPM)
and ventricular hypertrophy; X-rays showed pulmonary vascular congestion, and some pleural effusion (see insert).

The cause of Mrs. Bradford's congestive failure was thought
to be arteriosclerotic hypertensive disease. This was confirmed via arteriosclerotic changes on the eye grounds exam
and on angiography, her own history, and her family history.
Another supporting fact: At 168 pounds, she was markedly
overweight for her short (5 ft.) stature. Mrs. Bradford was
successfully treated with digitalis, a diuretic, and a 1500-
calorie, low-sodium diet.

All of this happened 14 years ago. Since then Mrs. Bradford
has come for regular checkups. At 76, she still enjoys remark-
ably good health for a woman of her years. She now weighs 138
pounds. Her X-ray shows normal heart size, and her lungs are
clear. Her heart rate has slowed to a normal 68, and she has no
more dyspnea or ankle edema. Most important to Mrs. Bradford, she can enjoy a good night's rest, and has the vitality for a
normal life.

Mrs. Bradford wisely sought medical help at an early stage
of CHF. Patients who delay develop later, more dramatic
signs: more rales, more distention of the neck veins, dullness
over the lower chest area due to pleural effusion, markedly
enlarged liver, and pitting ankle edema. (Bedridden patients
develop edema over the sacrum.)

Treatment commonplace

In all stages of congestive heart failure, treatment is relatively the same. It always includes:
- diuresis via low-sodium diet and diuretics
- semi-recumbent position for a day or two to drain edema and promote rest
- prevention of electrolyte imbalance
- digitalis to augment myocardial contractility.

If the patient has not taken digitalis before, a digitalizing dose is given the first day followed by maintenance doses. (So be sure to take an accurate drug history.)

In difficult cases, standard drug treatment may seem ineffective, and various drugs and dosages may need to be tried. In such cases, one of your most important tasks is accurate measurement of the daily weight, the best index of fluid status. Also monitor fluid intake, urine output, and vital signs. Auscultate the heart and lungs frequently for abnormal sounds (S_3, S_4, and rales). Notify the doctor if you find any change.

When patients do respond to treatment, congestive failure can come under satisfactory control in only a few days. Then the patient can resume normal life, continuing digitalis and diuretics with his doctor's supervision.

Throughout treatment, your nursing observations and care are crucial. Your observations begin at admission with baseline assessment of the patient's physical and mental status. This assessment should always include the patient's weight and vital signs: temperature, pulse, respirations, and blood pressure. Look at the patient. Observe his appearance, and take a thorough nursing history. Usually the complete history has to await a later time, since such patients are often in great distress when first hospitalized. But, the physical appearance, vital signs, and mental state are a mandatory baseline for measuring the effects of treatment.

Three stages of pulmonary edema

In its severest form, congestive heart failure causes pulmonary edema — an extreme emergency. Pulmonary edema almost always has its source in left ventricular failure that increases pressure in the pulmonary vascular bed and forces fluid and solutes from the intravascular compartment into the interstitium of the lungs (see insert, *A Closer Look at the Lungs*).

A closer look at the lungs
The lungs consist of three different anatomical entities which interconnect and influence each other. The first anatomical structure, the network of airways, consists of the trachea, major bronchi, small bronchial tubules, and alveoli. The second, or circulatory network, includes the pulmonary arteries, veins, arterioles, venules, and the capillary bed. These two networks are imbedded in the third, called the interstitium or interstitial space, which is composed of connective tissue.

The alveolar membranes and the pulmonary capillary membranes share a common basement membrane which facilitates the exchange of oxygen and carbon dioxide with the blood. The small alveolar vessels are chiefly involved in the function of gas exchange, while the extra-alveolar vessels and the lymphatics both help regulate fluid and solute movement within the interstitium. If the vascular compartment overloads with fluids, lymphatics ordinarily can drain away the excess.

Normally, the pressure in the pulmonary vascular bed is higher than in the surrounding interstitium. This pressure difference facilitates the movement of fluids out of the capillaries. However, solutes such as plasma proteins within capillaries exert serum colloid osmotic pressure which prevents too much fluid and electrolytes from leaving the vascular bed. Pulmonary edema can easily arise when this balance is disturbed.

1. *Interstitial stage*. Patients in this stage become short of breath with any exercise. They have difficulty climbing stairs. They can't sleep in a supine position because of dyspnea and spend whole nights sitting upright in a chair (orthopnea). They try to compensate by hyperventilating and so their PCO_2 falls while their PO_2 remains near or slightly below normal. They may complain of restlessness and a feeling of anxiety. During physical assessment of patients in this stage, you're likely to pick up an abnormal third heart sound, the diastolic gallop.

As the interstitium continues to swell with fluids, the lymphatic system can no longer handle the fluid overload. Fluid floods into the peripheral alveoli, further blocking adequate gas exchange. Now the patient's respiratory rate climbs and his auxiliary respiratory muscles begin to work. The increased respiratory effort uses up large amounts of oxygen, deepening the oxygen debt.

2. *Alveolar stage*. At this stage, both PO_2 and PCO_2 drop considerably below normal. As the PCO_2 falls, the pH rises. Hyperventilation blows off too much CO_2 and causes respiratory alkalosis. These rapid, labored respirations increase venous return to the heart, adding more venous blood to an already overloaded pulmonary capillary bed. Hypoxia increases and, in turn, triggers the release of catecholamines to stimulate cardiac action.

At this stage, an examiner can easily hear characteristic crepitant rales (bubbles of edema fluid mixed with surfactant, a lipid protein that coats the walls of the alveoli and keeps them from collapsing). When air goes through these fluid-filled alveoli, it makes this characteristic sound.

3. *Bronchial stage*. In the third stage, the small bronchioles begin to retain fluid. Now the bubbles are larger, and the sounds they make are not fine crepitant rales but coarse bubbling sounds. The bronchial tree tends to become spastic, causing the patient to wheeze. Such wheezing may cause the examiner to suspect asthma — hence this condition is sometimes called cardiac asthma.

As the bronchial tree fills with fluid, the patient's condition deteriorates. His arterial blood gas (ABG) studies show a sharp drop in PO_2. Tissues respond to the dwindling oxygen supply by resorting to anaerobic metabolism. This pours large quantities of lactic acid into the bloodstream, creating metabolic acidosis. The patient may begin wheezing and

MANAGING A PATIENT WITH PULMONARY EDEMA		
STAGES	SYMPTOMS	NURSING RESPONSIBILITIES
INITIAL	Persistent cough — patient feels "like a cold is coming on." Slight dyspnea/orthopnea Exercise intolerance Restlessness. Anxiety Crepitant rales may be heard over the dependent portion of the lungs Diastolic gallop.	Check color and amount of expectoration. Position patient for comfort. Auscultate chest for rales and third heart sound. Medicate as ordered. Monitor apical and radial pulses for rate and rhythm. Assist patient with all needs to conserve strength. Provide emotional support (through all stages) for patient and family.
ADVANCED	Acute shortness of breath Respirations — rapid noisy (audible wheeze, rales) Cough more intense and productive of frothy, blood-tinged sputum Cyanosis. Diaphoresis — skin cold and clammy Tachycardia — arrhythmias Hypotension.	Institute emergency measures: 1. Give oxygen — preferably by high concentration mask or IPPB. 2. Insert I.V. if not already done. 3. Aspirate nasopharynx p.r.n. 4. Apply rotating tourniquets. 5. Give digitalis and morphine as ordered. 6. Give potent diuretics (e.g., furosemide [Lasix] or ethacrynic acid [Edecrin]) as ordered. 7. Insert Foley catheter. 8. Calculate intake and output exactly. 9. Draw ABGs. 10. Attach cardiac monitor leads and observe EKG. 11. Prepare for phlebotomy, if necessary. 12. Have resuscitation equipment available.
ACUTE	Decreased level of consciousness Ventricular arrhythmias Shock Diminished breath sounds.	Give emotional support to patient and family. Be prepared for cardioversion of tachyarrhythmias. Assist with intubation and mechanical ventilation. Resuscitate if necessary.

cough up blood-tinged sputum. *His PCO_2 may start to level off, but don't mistake this for an improvement. It's a sign of incipient respiratory failure.*

In this final stage, pulmonary edema leaves the patient severely hypoxic and exhausted from nearly fruitless respiratory efforts. His PCO_2 rises markedly, and the combined sequelae of respiratory and metabolic acidosis put him in a precarious condition. Without immediate treatment, he'll die. Such treatment always includes diuretics, morphine, digitalis, and adequate oxygenation (see insert, *Managing a Patient with Pulmonary Edema*).

Mr. Stevens' case illustrates the details of such treatment. Less than 2 hours after calmly sitting down to watch his favorite television show, Mr. Stevens was in our emergency department...in acute distress. His skin felt cold and clammy, he had an elevated blood pressure, and he was cyanotic. His

Non-cardiac causes of P.E.
Conditions other than heart failure can cause pulmonary edema, such as:
- Toxins from infections or inhalants, and vasoactive substances, such as histamines, that increase capillary permeability, allow excess fluids into the lungs;
- Renal and hepatic diseases, and some nutritional disturbances that decrease serum colloid osmotic pressure, cause fluids to accumulate in the pulmonary interstitium;
- Diseases, such as Hodgkin's, that block normal lymphatic drainage, permit fluids to accumulate.

respirations sounded bubbly, with moist rales over both lungs. He had frothy, blood-tinged secretions in the corners of his mouth.

Mr. Stevens was in the final stage of respiratory failure from fulminating pulmonary edema. We quickly elevated his head, cleared his airway, then administered oxygen. He looked anxious and frightened, and became even more so as we hovered over him. A patient who fears that any moment he may stop breathing compounds his difficulties by expending more oxygen and producing more carbon dioxide than he would if he were calmer. So in low, confident tones, we continually explained what we were doing — why we were giving him oxygen, why we were starting an I.V., why we were repeatedly taking vital signs.

If a patient can cough and expectorate, he may be able to clear his airway. If he can't he'll need to be suctioned, as did Mr. Stevens. Once we'd made certain of an open airway and had drawn blood for an arterial blood gas analysis, we started him on high-concentration oxygen by mask. (The commonly used nasal cannula doesn't deliver enough oxygen to meet the needs of a patient with pulmonary edema.)

Mr. Stevens' initial ABG readings clearly showed that he was unable to maintain adequate ventilation on his own. With a pH of 7.0, a PCO_2 of 84, and a PO_2 of 64, he needed to be intubated immediately if we were to save his life. We quickly inserted an endotracheal tube and began ventilating him on an MA-1 respirator, FIO_2 100%. (Remember that oxygen must be administered in precisely prescribed doses or you risk over-oxygenating your patient. Avoid over-oxygenation by checking ABGs frequently and adjusting the ventilator accordingly. (see insert, *Checklist for Patients Receiving Oxygen*).

Mr. Stevens' respiratory acidosis was corrected quickly. His pH rose to 7.44 and his PCO_2 dropped to 32. However, despite the 100% oxygen, his PO_2 increased only to 96, meaning that much of his cardiac output was still being shunted past fluid-filled alveoli.

Drug regimen

To remove the excess alveolar fluid, we started I.V. diuretics with 40 mg of furosemide (Lasix). To keep track of his intake and output, we inserted a Foley catheter. Along with the diuretic, we gave Mr. Stevens an initial intravenous dose of

A CHECKLIST FOR PATIENTS RECEIVING OXYGEN

METHOD OF OXYGEN DELIVERY	FLOW RATE	PERCENTAGE OF OXYGEN DELIVERY (FIO$_2$)	PURPOSE OF TREATMENT	CAUTIONS
Nasal cannula	2-6 L/min	Up to 55%	Corrects hypoxia; decreases breathing efforts; lessens the work load of the heart.	Dries mucous membranes of nose and throat. Keep nasal passages clean.
Medium concentration mask	8-10 L/min (Never less than 5 L/min)	40%-70%	Same as above.	Fearing suffocation patients tolerate mask poorly. Keep face dry under mask to prevent irritation.
High concentration (non-rebreathing bag) mask	Sufficient to keep bag inflated. 6-10 L/min	60%-95%	Same as above.	Never allow bag to collapse completely during inspiration. Maintain a tight seal.
IPPB (Intermittent Positive Pressure Breathing)	Preset rate and volume	40%-80%	Decreases breathing efforts; improves patient's coughing mechanism; delivers bronchodilators; decreases venous return to heart; helps expand the lungs.	Discontinue treatment if hemoptysis occurs. Use temporarily in pulmonary edema. Contraindicated in pneumothorax without chest tube. Watch patient for tachycardia and dyspnea.
CMV (Continuous Mechanical Ventilation) Assist	Preset rate and volume	21%-100% as required	Augments patient's own ventilatory cycle; a determined amount of gas and oxygen is inspired.	Check ABGs frequently. Reassure and sedate patient as needed.
CMV (Continuous Mechanical Ventilation) Controlled	Preset rate and volume	21%-100% as required	Assumes total work of breathing.	Provide means for communication. Check settings.
CPAP (Continuous Positive Airway Pressure) Used on patient breathing spontaneously	Set as determined by patient's ABGs, age, and type of equipment used		Alleviates respiratory distress syndrome.	Check for decreasing cardiac output. Watch for pneumothorax.
PEEP (Positive End Expiratory Pressure) Used in intubated patients with suitable respirator or Ambu bag with PEEP valve	Same as above		Increases the lungs' functional residual capacity to its normal level (improves lung compliance); improves oxygenation without use of dangerously high oxygen concentration.	Hypotension may occur. Watch for signs of pneumothorax.

morphine, 4 mg. and deslanoside (Cedilanid D), 0.8 mg. Digitalis strengthens cardiac contractions and increases cardiac output while slowing the heart rate. These effects benefit patients whose pulmonary edema is secondary to cardiac problems. But digitalis must be used cautiously.

Morphine is essential. It alleviates the extreme anxiety of the patient who is literally drowning in his own secretions. It also reduces the tremendous work of breathing and decreases peripheral vascular resistance, so more blood remains in the dilated peripheral vascular bed. But even when given slowly, morphine can severely depress respiration, so keep handy a supply of naloxone (Narcan) and intubation equipment. Avoid giving morphine to patients with a history of cerebrovascular accident, chronic obstructive pulmonary disease, or cardiogenic shock.

Fortunately, Mr. Stevens recovered sufficiently with repeated doses of diuretics and digitalis. After 24 hours, he no longer needed ventilatory assistance. If he had not responded, other treatments could have been added (such as nitroprusside [Nipride] to reduce afterload). Aminophylline may help dilate bronchi and increase cardiac output. (But give this drug slowly to prevent a sudden — possibly fatal — drop in blood pressure.) Sodium bicarbonate may also be ordered for severe metabolic acidosis.

You can reduce the amount of circulating blood by rotating tourniquets to keep it pooled in the extremities. This diminishes venous return and concentrates the heart's energy on circulating blood in the head and trunk where it's needed most. But check radial and pedal pulses frequently, making certain that tourniquets haven't stopped circulation to the extremities entirely. Remember, explain to the patient on tourniquets that his arms and legs will be temporarily discolored during treatment. At the end of the procedure, remember to remove one tourniquet at a time to prevent a sudden rush of blood to the heart. Phlebotomy sometimes helps (if the patient is not anemic) by decreasing circulatory load and reducing the heart's work. Check vital signs frequently during the procedure, which simply involves draining 500 to 700 ml of blood, under sterile conditions. As Mr. Stevens' case shows, pulmonary edema can develop suddenly and dramatically. If you know how to intervene quickly and correctly, your service to the patient can be lifesaving.

Cardiac Complications
Often catastrophic

BY SALLY A. BOWERS, RN

ONCE A PATIENT WITH severe cardiac dysfunction has been admitted to a coronary care unit, his chances of survival are reasonably good — unless he develops certain complications. To detect these complications before they become catastrophic, you must know: what these complications are; what you can do to prevent them; how to detect them in their earliest, most treatable stages; and what the appropriate treatment is so you can give it promptly.

The major complications are these: cardiogenic shock, ventricular aneurysm, and cardiac tamponade.

Cardiogenic shock — most perilous

Cardiogenic shock is now the major complication leading to death in patients with myocardial infarction. Ten to 15% of patients with MI develop cardiogenic shock; their mortality rate is 85% or greater.

How to recognize it? Usually, the patient in cardiogenic shock has cold, clammy skin and a systolic blood pressure below 80 mm Hg. But don't be fooled by an initially normal blood pressure. Hypertensive patients may drop their blood pressure 20 to 30 mm Hg and still have a systolic pressure over

The Swan-Ganz catheter

The most reliable index of left ventricular function is the left ventricular end diastolic pressure (LVEDP), obtained with a Swan-Ganz catheter (see page 105). When pumping is insufficient, left ventricular blood volume and then the LVEDP, left atrial pressure (LAP), pulmonary arterial pressure (PAP), and pulmonary wedge pressures (PWP) can all rise. The normal pressures? LVEDP, 12 mm Hg or less; PAP, 25/10 mm Hg; and PWP, 4 to 12 mm Hg. In cardiogenic shock, you're likely to see a pulmonary artery wedge pressure greater than 15 mm Hg due to left ventricular failure.

Closely monitor the EKG while the doctor inserts the Swan-Ganz. Have Lidocaine and a defibrillator handy. Once the catheter is in place, monitor the PAP continuously. Keep the line patent with a pressurized, heparinized flush solution.

If you get a poor pressure tracing, check to make sure all connections are tight, stopcocks are turned in the right direction; the catheter hasn't kinked; there are no air bubbles in the tubing or connections; and the balloon is deflated. A damped tracing may indicate that the catheter is clotting, or that the catheter may not be in the correct position. Try to aspirate the clot and flush the catheter, but not unless the clot can be withdrawn or the catheter can be pulled back 5 cm. Avoid using the catheter to draw blood samples, for this increases the chance of clotting within the catheter.

Use the PA line for pressure readings only, not as another I.V. line for medications. To avoid the need to reposition the catheter, make sure it's firmly secured to the patient's chest so it won't be pulled out of place inadvertently.

90. Other symptoms include pallor, cyanosis, mental confusion or obtundation, and urine output less than 20 ml per hour.

Watch for subtle changes in the patient's sensorium — they may be your first clue to impending shock. You'd expect a patient who has suffered a heart attack to be concerned and anxious. But *undue* restlessness and confusion should make you suspect poor cerebral vascular perfusion from a falling cardiac output. A patient in this situation can quickly deteriorate into coma.

Another result of decreased cardiac output is overall hypoxemia. Consequently, the arterial blood gas determinations in patients with cardiogenic shock show a markedly depressed PO_2. This hypoxemia can cause metabolic (lactic) acidosis and low pH. You must correct such acidosis promptly, since it further weakens myocardial function and may make the heart refractory to certain drugs, particularly the vasopressors.

Systolic blood pressure usually falls before *diastolic,* so you may notice a narrowing pulse pressure. If the patient is hypertensive, consider a drop to 100 mm Hg, or to 40 mm Hg below baseline level, definite hypotension. When such hypotension accompanies oliguria (urine output below 20 ml per hour) and other signs of diminished cardiac output (cyanosis and confusion), cardiogenic shock is probably present. Urine output falls because inadequate kidney perfusion activates the renin-angiotensin system to release angiotensin, an active vasopressor. At the same time, increased aldosterone stimulates the kidney to retain sodium and water.

Once you're sure hypotension is present, rule out possible causes of precipitous fall in blood pressure: pain, excessive analgesia, hypoxemia, arrhythmias, trinitrates, and antihypertensive drugs. If you suspect shock, remember that tachycardia and bradycardia can cause a shock-like syndrome, but its symptoms are reversible once arrhythmia is corrected. So, if the patient has tachycardia or bradycardia, antiarrhythmic treatment alone may boost cardiac output.

Rule out extracardiac causes

Quickly evaluate possible extracardiac causes for shock so that appropriate treatment can begin. For example, hypoxia from extracardiac (respiratory) causes may impair cardiac function; in such cases, improving respiration reverses shock.

Port for
inflating
balloon

Thermistor

Port for
measuring CVP

Port for measuring
PAP and PWP

Similarly, pain may cause a vasovagal response mimicking shock; effective analgesia will counteract it. Morphine and myocardial antiarrhythmic drugs can decrease cardiac output and blood pressure. So, evaluate their effects carefully as another possible cause of shock. If shock persists after all these factors have been eliminated or treated, evaluate central venous pressure (CVP), or, more reliably, the left ventricular end-diastolic pressure (LVEDP) (see page 104). If the pulmonary arterial pressure is low or normal, begin treatment to expand blood volume.

Treatment
Treatment of cardiogenic shock aims to increase blood pressure and coronary artery perfusion and thereby improve cardiac function. Specifically, such treatment should increase cardiac output and preserve ischemic myocardium by decreasing preload (related to LVEDP), afterload (stress in the ventricular wall during muscle shortening), and myocardial oxygen consumption. Treatment usually begins with intravenous infusions to expand blood volume, if hypovolemia is present. Hypovolemia can result from many things such as

Four ways to measure
Doctors use this Swan-Ganz Thermodilution catheter — a quadruple-lumen catheter inserted into the right heart — to measure cardiac output, CVP, pulmonary artery pressure, and pulmonary wedge pressure. One port contains a thermistor tip to which the cardiac output monitor is connected.

Nursing actions for IABP problems

Thrombus formation due to blood cells clumping around balloon or decreased blood flow in affected limb: Check perfusion in extremities; watch for CVA; administer I.V. heparin carefully as ordered; check clotting times daily.

Hemorrhage or thrombocytopenia due to platelet destruction by IABP and anticoagulant therapy: Check dressings over arterial lines, Swan-Ganz, pacemaker, and IABP insertion site for bleeding qlh; order daily CBC and clotting studies (platelet count will decrease slightly in patient on heparin and IABP); administer packed cells and platelets as ordered.

Volume depletion and anemia due to too many blood samples: Tell doctor how much blood work is being done.

Lower perfusion to renal arteries and left arm due to balloon displacement: Check urine volume and specific gravity qlh; check balloon position on X-ray; check perfusion to extremities.

IABP malfunction due to poor triggering from arrhythmias: Treat

(continued, opposite page)

excessive diuresis, rigid fluid restriction, emesis from digitalis toxicity, hemorrhages and subcutaneous hematomas (after anticoagulants), or prolonged use of vasopressors.

If the PA wedge pressure is less than 15 mm Hg, you can try a fluid challenge — usually with rapid infusion of salt-poor albumin (100 ml in 10 to 15 minutes). But crystalline solutions, such as saline or dextrose in water, may also be used. In either case, this therapy is hazardous, so monitor it carefully. Record baseline pressures before the infusion starts; measure them again in the middle and at the end of the infusion. Make sure I.V. lines are patent and avoid interstitial infiltration. Consider fluid infusion helpful if blood pressure and urine output improve without a rapid rise in pulmonary wedge pressure. However, if you find pulmonary rales and congestion, discontinue the infusion immediately. If arterial pressure does not improve after the infusion (that is, systolic remains below 90 mm Hg) and if urine output remains below 20 ml/hour, the doctor will add drug treatment to improve cardiac function.

Cardiac drugs

Such treatment might include intravenous dopamine, which in small doses may not significantly increase myocardial oxygen demands. Dopamine dilates all vascular beds, increases mesenteric and renal blood flow, and improves cardiac output by decreasing afterload and preload.

What's the dosage? Usually, an ampul of dopamine (5 ml/ 200 mg) is diluted in 250 to 500 ml of a dextrose or saline solution. It's infused at a rate of 5 to 30 mcg/kg/minute (or maximum 50 mcg/kg/minute). Whenever possible, infuse dopamine into a large vein to avoid extravasation with necrosis and sloughing of surrounding tissue. Dopamine is best given with an infusion pump or microdrip regulator to avoid an inadvertent bolus and gross fluctuations in blood pressure.

During dopamine infusion, monitor for sinus tachycardia or atrial or ventricular arrhythmias. Such arrhythmias may occur at the beginning of dopamine infusion, but usually subside after 15 to 20 minutes. If they persist (or if blood pressure does not improve), dopamine may have to be discontinued and another drug substituted. Norepinephine is sometimes used. It does increase the rate and force of myocardial contraction, but has the disadvantage of increasing oxygen demand. Most doctors avoid giving isoproterenol because it shunts cardiac output to nonvital areas (skin and skeletal muscle). And it decreases oxygen supply to the myocardium by lowering diastolic perfusion pressure.

When a vasopressor can maintain blood pressure above 90 to 100 mm Hg, concomitant use of a vasodilator (nitroprusside, Nipride), further improves cardiac output by reducing afterload (as it lowers aortic systolic pressure). Far more potent and shorter acting than the nitrates, nitroprusside relaxes both arteries and veins. It takes effect very rapidly (within minutes). So monitor carefully for tachycardia, ventricular arrhythmias, or falling blood pressure. Do not allow blood pressure to drop below 80 mm Hg. If blood pressure falls to this level, stop the infusion. Nitroprusside is light-sensitive, so cover the solution bag and infusion lines with nontransparent paper or foil. Discard any solution after 4 hours, since the drug loses potency after that time.

Give analgesics as needed if the patient is conscious and in pain, since this itself can cause hypotension.

Take samples for blood-gas determinations every 4 hours to see that the PO_2 stays higher than 75 mm Hg. The patient may need oxygen therapy or intubation and mechanical ventilation for adequate oxygen exchange. He may also need sodium bicarbonate to correct metabolic acidosis.

Circulatory assist will be needed next if, after treatment, cardiac output is less than 2 liters per minute; if systolic pressure is less than 80 mm Hg (or 100 mm Hg in a previously hypertensive patient); or if urinary output is less than 20 ml per hour.

Help for the failing heart
The intra-aortic balloon pump (IABP) is commonly used to increase coronary perfusion and assist the failing heart by decreasing its workload. It can sometimes save lives of patients with cardiogenic shock.

The balloon catheter is a thin-walled pumping chamber. It gets introduced into one of the femoral arteries (whichever one has the stronger pulse) and passed up the aorta into a position just distal to the left subclavian artery. Inflation of the balloon gets triggered by the patient's own EKG. It inflates during ventricular diastole (displacing blood proximally and increasing blood flow to the coronary arteries). It deflates before systole, before the aortic valve opens, allowing the ventricle to

arrhythmias as ordered; for sinus tachycardia (110 BPM) use a 2:1 trigger; for supraventricular tachycardia, try cardioversion or drugs; use external pacing for bradycardia or to override accelerated rhythm.

Diastolic augmentation below optimum: To determine reason for reduced augmentation, check arterial line patency, kinks in IABP catheter, bend in affected limb, need to refill balloon with carbon dioxide or helium, position of balloon, and timing adjustments.

Restricted mobility due to many lines and catheters: Use passive and active exercises for limbs as tolerated; turn and position patient, but don't elevate his head more than 30°, due to balloon location; avoid sharp flexion of the leg.

Sleep deprivation, disorientation, or denial in conscious patient: Explain equipment and procedures carefully; plan continuity of care, using same staff members each shift, if possible; use medications to promote relaxation and emotional stability, if condition permits.

Always keep an IABP machine set on automatic alarm.

When not to wean

Discontinue weaning a patient from an intra-aortic balloon pump if any of the following physical signs develop:
- Hypotension
- Increased pulmonary wedge pressure (PWP)
- Decreased urine output
- Clouding sensorium
- Angina
- S-T or T wave changes indicating ischemia
- Arrhythmias (PVCs) or change in heart rate.

contract against lower pressure and decreasing the afterload.

A cardiovascular surgeon usually inserts the balloon catheter at bedside and confirms its position on chest film. The balloon should be distal to the left subclavian artery in the thoracic aorta. Change the dressings over the balloon insertion site daily, using sterile technique. And watch for signs of infection.

Monitor constantly for hemodynamic changes. In case of ventricular fibrillation or cardiac arrest, turn the balloon pump off during external cardiac massage to prevent injury to the heart (see page 113). It's possible to coordinate chest compression with automatic balloon inflation and deflation, but the precise timing needed is difficult to maintain in an emergency situation.

Consider the response to IABP satisfactory if....
- blood pressure rises
- urinary output increases
- the patient is alert
- CVP and pulmonary arterial wedge pressures are normal
- vasopressors are no longer needed.

The patient can then be weaned from the balloon. How? By gradually decreasing the volume of gas inflating the balloon, or by decreasing the ratio at which the balloon inflates (1:2 to 1:6).

But if there's been no circulatory improvement (see insert above), the patient may be continued on the balloon (as long as several weeks) or evaluated for surgery. For example, arteriography can be done with the balloon in place to check the extent of infarction and coronary artery occlusion. Depending on the findings, the patient may need coronary bypass or resection of the ventricular wall (infarctectomy). Unfortunately, most patients in cardiogenic shock are too sick to make surgery feasible.

Mr. Levinthal's case illustrates the complexities of treating cardiogenic shock.

Mr. Levinthal, a 58-year-old foreman, was hospitalized with acute inferior wall myocardial infarction. He had a history of hypertension and an earlier myocardial infarction. At admission, his blood pressure was 130/85; pulse 110, sinus; respirations 34. He had severe chest pain and pulmonary edema. We quickly established an I.V. with 5% dextrose in water and gave nasal oxygen at 4L/min. We gave morphine sulphate, 4 mg, and furosemide (Lasix), 40 mg, (both intravenously), and

Pump position
This illustration shows an intra-aortic balloon pump in place.

Intra-aortic balloon

Balloon insertion via femoral artery

applied rotating tourniquets. We inserted a urinary catheter which drained 200 ml of urine. Over the next several hours, Mr. Levinthal's BP fell to 80/50; his pulse rate rose to 120; his respirations to 36. He became increasingly lethargic and the doctor suspected cardiogenic shock. An isoproterenol (Isuprel) infusion was begun (1 mg in 500 ml of 5% dextrose in water).

At this point, Mr. Levinthal was semiconscious and profoundly cyanotic. His blood pressure was 100/70 mm Hg; PCO_2, 32 mm Hg; PO_2, 56 mm Hg and pH, 7.28. An EKG showed sinus tachycardia with occasional unifocal PVCs. For the previous 2 hours, his urine output had been only 10 ml. The doctor decided to intubate and placed Mr. Levinthal on a ventilator with FIO_2 at 60%. On the ventilator, Mr. Levinthal's PO_2 rose to 78 mm Hg, PCO_2 was 36 mm Hg; and pH, 7.31. He was given an ampul (50 ml-44 mEq) of sodium bicarbonate and his FIO_2 raised to 70%. He remained barely conscious.

A Swan-Ganz catheter was inserted. His PA mean pressure was 30 mm Hg; cardiac output was 2.9 L/minute. An intra-arterial catheter was inserted in his left radial artery, and preparations made for insertion of an intra-aortic balloon (IABP). The Isuprel infusion was stopped and dopamine (Intropin) begun at the rate of 20 mcg/kg/minute. Blood pressure remained low at around 95/70. Urine output improved slightly in the next hour to 20 ml/hour.

A 45-ml balloon catheter was inserted through the left femoral artery, and 1:1 diastolic augmentation began. His heart rate at this time was 118 and augmentation was inadequate. So counterpulsation was raised to a 1:2 ratio. This worked much better. Mr. Levinthal improved slightly, and his urine output rose to 25 ml/hour. His heart rate came down to 100, so the balloon ratio was set back to a 1:1 ratio with better response. PO_2 remained around 85 mm Hg and pH improved to 7.37. At this time, mean PA was 26 mm Hg.

Mr. Levinthal was receiving digoxin 0.25 mg daily, and heparin 2000 units I.V. q2h. On the 4th day on IABP, he needed lidocaine infusion for multi-focal PVCs but these subsided without recurrence. Dopamine was gradually withdrawn and discontinued on the 5th day of IABP. His vital signs remained fairly stable.

By the 7th day on IABP, Mr. Levinthal was weaned from the ventilator to oxygen by face mask at FIO_2, 50%. His BP was

110/60 with augmented diastolic pressure of 110 mm Hg. Heart rate was stable at 95 to 100, respiration, 26. He was slightly confused and disoriented. Blood gas determinations remained good. But Mr. Levinthal was still balloon-dependent. Weaning began on the 9th day of IABP with 1:2 augmentation ratio. He continued to improve and was transferred out of CCU a week later.

Some advances have been made in treating cardiogenic shock, but the main goal is still prevention by early detection of pump failure. Recent investigations have examined the theory that pump failure actually results from the infarction itself and the inflammatory and chemical changes that flow from it. For example, we know that the amines released in response to the occlusion cause most of the damage that follows (tissue destruction and clot formation). Experiments are now being done with drugs such as hyaluronidase, anti-inflammatory drugs, and thrombolytic agents to see if they can prevent extension of infarction. This seems to be the most promising direction for decreasing mortality in cardiogenic shock.

Ventricular aneurysm: Risk of embolism

When massive infarction destroys a large section of left ventricle, the necrotic muscle can be reduced to a thin layer of fibrous tissue. When this thin layer dilates under the high pressure from the ventricular wall, it forms a separate noncontractile sac. Such an aneurysm is common in the anterior portion of the left ventricle (the area supplied by the anterior descending coronary artery), but may also occur posteriorly. Depending on size, you can see such an aneurysm on X-ray, as a definite bulge in the left ventricle.

In patients with ventricular aneurysm, stasis within the aneurysm can cause mural thrombi and systemic embolization. So, check peripheral pulses regularly, as well as the color and temperature of the extremities. Also, watch for changes in sensorium that may herald a CVA.

What confirms a suspected ventricular aneurysm? Several tests can confirm it: echocardiography, radioisotopic myocardial imaging, and ventriculography at cardiac catheterization. Coronary arteriography can pinpoint such an aneurysm. But it's contraindicated for 2 to 3 months after an acute MI.

Most patients who undergo resection of a ventricular aneurysm simultaneously have coronary bypass graft (see

Aneurysm in the ventricle
A severe heart attack that destroys a large section of the left ventricle can produce a ventricular aneurysm like the one here. Necrotic tissue reduces to a thin sheath of fibrous tissue. High pressure in the ventricular wall causes this tissue to dilate. It then becomes a noncontractile sac, separate from the ventricle.

Most aneurysms are located in the anterior portion of the left ventricle, an area supplied by the anterior descending coronary artery. But they can be found in the posterior portion as well.

Depending on the size, you may be able to see an aneurysm on a chest X-ray. If it's visible, you'll see a suspicious bulge in the area of the left ventricle. A patient with a ventricular aneurysm may have persistent tachycardia, intractable heart failure, and anginal pain that doesn't abate with nitrates.

Chapter 7). Without such resection, their prognosis depends on prevention of subsequent infarctions and congestive heart failure. Ventricular aneurysm can sometimes enlarge, but this is extremely rare.

Cardiac tamponade: Extreme emergency

Any fluid or blood in the pericardium limits ventricular ability to fill during diastole. If 150 to 200 ml of blood accumulates quickly in this closed membranous sac, it's a medical emergency — cardiac tamponade. The ventricle is so compressed that it can't eject forcefully, cardiac output falls, and the patient dies as the ventricle becomes too small to fill.

You'll see tamponade most often after open-heart surgery. Rarely, you'll see it after ventricular rupture, a complication of MI: When it occurs, it usually does so in the first week after infarction. Its cause is not well understood. There are usually no warning signs. A large perforation is, of course, immediately fatal. Sometimes, a smaller one leaves enough circulation to sustain a patient until he can get to the operating room for surgical repair. The clinical signs of cardiac tamponade may include falling blood pressure and shock syndrome, a rise in CVP, increased jugular vein distention, cyanosis, pulsus paradoxus, and faint heart sounds.

A conscious patient may describe such a slow perforation as a sharp or tearing pain over the precordium (not substernal, like angina). He reports that such pain varies with posture or respiration. In patients with such slow perforations, X-rays may show an enlarging cardiac shadow before clinical signs develop, but this is rare. Almost always, the onset of tamponade is sudden and catastrophic.

Cardiac tamponade needs immediate relief via pericardiocentesis or sternotomy. If the patient can't be moved to an O.R., sternotomy may be performed at the bedside using a thoracotomy tray. Have sterile equipment and blood available for rapid transfusion. Assemble emergency resuscitation equipment, including sterile internal defibrillator paddles at the bedside. Monitor the patient's EKG, CVP, and arterial pressure. There's usually no time for chest X-rays before sternotomy unless the tamponade has had a slow onset. However, as a temporary medical treatment (before pericardiocentesis or sternotomy can be done), simple intravenous infusion of fluid can be lifesaving. A rapid I.V. infusion

Success with CPR

External cardiac massage and artificial ventilation must begin within 4 to 6 minutes after cardiac arrest or irreversible brain damage will develop. To perform cardiopulmonary resuscitation (CPR) properly, you must receive instruction from a qualified instructor. These pictures merely illustrate the four basic steps of life support:

1. If the patient is unconscious, tilt his head back to relieve tongue obstruction and open his airway.

2. If he doesn't breathe spontaneously, begin artificial ventilation using a mouth-to-mouth or mouth-to-nose technique. Deliver several full breaths in quick succession.

3. Check his carotid artery for a pulse. If his neck is injured, feel instead for a femoral pulse.

4. If you can't feel a pulse, begin CPR immediately. Establish the correct position, and begin downward compressions, depressing the sternum 1½ to 2 inches. Maintain a rhythm of 80 compressions per minute if you are alone and 60 per minute if you are working with someone else.

Consider resuscitation efforts effective if you observe the following signs:
- constriction of the pupils
- carotid and femoral pulsations with each cardiac compression
- blinking upon stimulation of the eyelid
- breathing that begins spontaneously
- movement and struggling
- decreased cyanosis.

may allow the ventricle to fill enough to maintain reasonable cardiac output until the surgeon comes. So, if you suspect cardiac tamponade, start an I.V. infusion of 5% dextrose in water immediately.

During sternotomy, the mediastinum is cleared of blood and clots, allowing the ventricle full space for expansion and contraction. The patient's improvement is dramatic: immediate decrease in CVP, rise in blood pressure, and disappearance of cyanosis. After the sternum is closed, the patient should have prophylactic antibiotics.

Postoperatively, such patients need meticulous care of chest tubes. For the first several hours, you must milk and drain the chest tubes every 15 minutes to prevent clots from blocking drainage. Also, record the amount drained, noting whether it is sanguineous or serosanguineous. Report any sudden tachycardia, unexplained hypotension or sudden cessation of chest drainage to the doctor. Keep a Fogarty catheter handy to unclog a chest drain.

Pericardiocentesis is no less dangerous. Its risks include sudden death by laceration of a coronary artery or ventricular fibrillation, so keep emergency drugs and resuscitation equipment available. A large-bore needle is introduced into the pericardium through the skin to the left of the xiphoid process. An EKG lead attached to this needle identifies contact with the heart surface, decreasing the chance of injury to the myocardium. Repeated aspirations may be necessary and the patient may still need surgery to complete the evacuation.

After pericardiocentesis, watch for arrhythmias such as PVCs that may follow needle trauma.

Cardiac tamponade is a potentially reversible complication, if it's recognized immediately and intervention is available.

Inflammatory Heart Diseases
Four most common

BY MARY M. CANOBBIO, RN, BSN

INFLAMMATORY DISEASES of the heart were once nearly always lethal. Antibiotics have made them much less so and, in fact, much less prevalent. But they do still occur. They still produce life-threatening changes in the heart muscle and its structures — changes that are often difficult to recognize and to treat. To improve your own ability to deal with inflammatory diseases of the heart, you may want to review the most common ones: myocarditis, bacterial endocarditis, pericarditis, and rheumatic heart disease.

Myocarditis
Myocarditis denotes an infiltration of the myocardial cells by bacteria or viruses. These pathogens can cause myocardial damage by inciting toxic reactions or inflammatory response.

Myocarditis can occur after infection with almost any pathogen. For example, infection with group B-Coxsackie virus can induce myocarditis in neonates and infants. Some pathogens that can induce myocarditis include: bacteria *(Clostridium diphtheriae, S. pneumoniae);* viruses *(Coxsackie group B);* protozoas *(Trypanosoma cruzi,* the major cause of Chagas' diseases in South America); and fungi *(His-*

Pathology of myocarditis

In myocarditis, myocardial fibers disintegrate and diffuse throughout the myocardium, along with infiltrated lymphocytes. Certain pathogens, usually bacteria, may form localized microabscesses in the interstitium; viruses directly cause inflammation and necrosis of the myocardium. Toxins such as the endotoxin of typhoid fever, may also produce inflammation as an allergic response. These changes may be localized or widespread.

Because they are susceptible to myocarditis, patients with rheumatic heart disease should receive prophylactic antibiotics before dental, genitourinary, and obstetric procedures. Also watch for such inflammation in patients with indwelling catheters. To prevent it, use aseptic technique when giving catheter care.

toplasma capsulatum or *candida*). But infections are not the only cause of myocarditis. Secondary causes of myocarditis include rheumatic fever and other diseases that produce myocardial inflammation (such as bacterial endocarditis).

What symptoms?

During the acute phase, the symptoms are systemic: fever, malaise, arthralgias, and fatigue. The patient may also have precordial discomfort typical of pericarditis or of angina. Other symptoms vary according to the extent of myocardial infiltration and may include tachycardia (unrelated to fever), hypotension, and symptoms of congestive failure. On auscultation, you may find a soft first heart sound, gallop rhythm, or systolic murmur (suggesting ventricular dilatation and mitral regurgitation). EKGs may show conduction disturbance (particularly prolonged P-R interval and ST-T wave changes), but these are often nonspecific for myocarditis.

Treatment of myocarditis includes bedrest during the acute stages and management of symptoms with: diuretics, digitalis, and salt restriction for heart failure; and, antiarrhythmics as needed (which call for careful monitoring). Patients with viral myocarditis are very sensitive to digitalis and should have the short-acting forms, such as digoxin (Lanoxin). Generally, your nursing care is the same as that for any patient with an acute infection or congestive heart failure. Check for signs of cardiovascular deterioration. Assess breath sounds, vital signs, and central venous pressures frequently. Watch urine output. Report an output less than 30 ml/hr to the doctor. Also report any weight gain (worsening edema).

Bacterial endocarditis

Endocarditis means an acute or subacute (SBE/subacute bacterial endocarditis) bacterial (or fungal) invasion of the endothelial heart muscle and heart valves. Endocarditis is usually classified by the causative organism and clinical findings. Acute endocarditis is usually attributed to *Staphylococcus aureus* or *Pneumoccoccus*; subacute bacterial endocarditis (SBE), to *Streptococcus viridans*.

Endocardial pathogens may enter via the skin, respiratory, gastrointestinal, or genitourinary tracts. These pathogens take hold most easily in patients with lowered endocardial resistance (patients with infections after congenital or rheumatic heart disease, or those recovering from open heart surgery, especially if they have prosthetic valve replacement and a history of drug abuse). It's crucial to use aseptic technique when changing surgical dressings. Patients with normal valves who have been infected via dental sepsis (*Streptococcus viridans* is common in the mouth) tend to be unusually vulnerable to bacterial infection in general. Who gets bacterial endocarditis? Mostly young adults with a history of rheumatic fever, and some children with congenital heart defects.

Endocardial pathogens typically settle on the cardiac valves (often the mitral or aortic). Characteristically, they first infiltrate the contact aspect of the cusps but eventually extend through their full thickness. These bacterial colonies multiply by platelet and fibrin aggregation and set up an inflammatory vegetative process. Eventually these bulky vegetations prevent proper alignment of the valve cusps, producing poor closure and incompetence. The result may be scarring, retraction of leaflets, and ensuing insufficiency. These vegetations also have a tendency to dislodge and embolize.

Symptoms sometimes specific

The patient with endocarditis has a history of chronic fever — usually low-grade and intermittent. Depending on the virulence of the organism involved, he may also have nocturnal sweats and chills, malaise, easy fatigue, anorexia, or arthralgia. These nonspecific symptoms often lead to studies for "fever of unknown origin," unless certain diagnostic findings (petechiae, Osler's nodes, splinter hemorrhages over nail beds, systolic murmurs [a sign of aortic stenosis or mitral regurgitation], and splenomegaly) point clearly to bacterial endocarditis. In elderly patients, a CVA with fever due to cerebral embolus from an infected valve may be the *first* sign of endocarditis.

What laboratory findings to expect? Blood cultures are positive for pathogens in 80 to 90% of patients. Other laboratory findings include an elevated sedimentation rate (90%) with slight leukocytosis and anemia (in SBE). Echocardiograms help to evaluate the extent of valvular damage. Electrocardiograms are generally not diagnostically helpful; but certain arrhythmias (such as atrial fibrillation) do point to valvular disease. Since none of these tests is specific for bacterial endocarditis, an accurate medical (and dental) history is

Signs of bacterial endocarditis
Endocarditis often produces a persistent low-grade fever, fatigue, and anorexia that may be mistaken for symptoms of flu. Certain physical findings of bacterial endocarditis, however, can help pinpoint the correct diagnosis:
● Petechiae usually found in the oral mucosa, conjunctiva, upper chest, and lower extremities
● Tender, raised erythematous lesions found on the fingers and toe pads, known as Osler's nodes
● Non-tender splinter hemorrhages over the nail beds, as seen above
● Systolic murmurs, a sign of mitral or aortic regurgitation, which occur in 85% of these cases
● Pain in the left upper quadrant due to splenomegaly.

Dangerous growth
This drawing shows the growth of vegetations that is characteristic of endocarditis. These vegetations, composed of fibrin, red cells, and platelets, settle most commonly on the aortic and mitral valves and can dislodge, causing life-threatening emboli.

crucial for diagnosis.

Major complications of endocarditis include: emboli from dislodged vegetations (which predispose to vascular accidents); nephritis, renal infarcts, and uremia; and heart failure (from severe valvular damage). Vital signs are the earliest clue to complications, so watch for changes in the temperature and respirations, and monitor the apical pulse to detect changes in heart rhythm and rate.

Managing endocarditis
Patients hospitalized with endocarditis are often very sick at admission. Typically, they are dehydrated and anorexic, and show severe weight loss. They may need parenteral fluids. Because they have fever, remember to encourage oral fluid intake, too. Also keep track of their nutritional state; offer frequent small meals — likely to be more acceptable than large ones. Finally, remember that these patients need emotional support since their illness requires long-term hospitalization. As they begin to feel less acutely ill, they tend to become bored, depressed, angry and frustrated; they need special support at such times.

Treatment aims to eradicate the infection; prevent cardiac damage and complications; treat the cardiac problems due to the inflammation; replace damaged valves when indicated; and finally, prevent spread or recurrence of infection.

Eradicating the infection obviously requires identification of the infecting pathogen, followed by appropriate antibiotic treatment. Endocarditis after penicillinase-producing staphylococcal infection calls for a penicillinase-resistant antibiotic given intravenously over a 6 to 8 week period. Such drugs include: methicillin (Staphcillin) 16-20 g/day; oxacillin (Prostaphlin) 4-6 g/day; or cephalothin (Keflin) 10-14 g/day. If the pathogen is *Streptococcus viridans*, or a non-penicillinase-producing staphylococcus, the best drug is intravenous penicillin-G potassium (usual dose in adults, 10 to 12 million units daily for 4 to 6 weeks). Remember to watch the serum potassium level in patients who need large doses of penicillin-G potassium. Such patients need routine assessment of renal function (BUN and creatinine). For patients allergic to penicillin, cephalothin (Keflin) and vancomycin (Vancocin) are effective substitutes. Some patients allergic to penicillin are also allergic to the cephalosporins.

In 10 to 20% of patients with endocarditis, blood cultures come up negative even in repeated tests. Such patients may receive aqueous penicillin-G, 12-20 million units daily I.V., for 4 weeks, with streptomycin, 1 g daily, during the first 10 days of treatment.

Preventing cardiac damage and complications depends almost entirely on early diagnosis and treatment. Unfortunately, many patients go untreated for a long time, until progressive weakness, persistent fever, and general malaise force them to seek help. When finally hospitalized, they are usually quite debilitated, and dehydrated, and have some signs of cardiac complications. Watch for early signs of cardiac involvement: irregular pulse, tachycardia, chest discomfort, dyspnea on exertion, and any signs of heart failure and emboli. To help such patients recover, monitor their activity and promote plenty of rest; see that bedridden patients are turned frequently; teach coughing and deep-breathing exercises, and provide antiembolic stockings. Auscultate breath sounds carefully to detect early signs of failure or secondary respiratory infections.

Preventing recurring infection requires prophylactic use of

Valve replacement
Here you can see a prosthetic
Starr Edwards mitral valve in
place.

antibiotics during procedures known to cause bacteremia in high-risk patients. Such patients include those with congenital heart lesions, rheumatic fever, known valvular disease, or cardiac murmurs. They need prophylactic antibiotics and special care during any procedures likely to cause transient bacteremia (dental work and any genitourinary or gastrointestinal procedures). They should seek medical treatment for persistent sore throats or any bacterial infection like boils on the skin.

When cardiac problems persist

What if, despite antibiotic therapy, the patient continues to show signs of cardiac failure, valvular damage, deteriorating cardiac function or persistent bacteremia? Then he may need evaluation for surgical correction (such as prosthetic replacement of the mitral or aortic valves). Whenever possible, surgery is deferred until after the sepsis is controlled. The decision for surgery is often difficult because these patients are typically poor surgical risks — especially when they are elderly, or have heart failure, or severely incompetent valves. Consider Mr. Jarvis.

Mr. Jacob Jarvis, a 31-year-old jeweler, was hospitalized for treatment of subacute bacterial endocarditis. He had been treating himself at home for what he thought was the flu. At admission, he had fever, dyspnea, and general malaise. Physical exam revealed a Grade III/VI systolic murmur at the apex, with engorged neck veins and bilateral rales over the lung fields. He had scattered petechiae on his upper chest; he did not have Osler's nodes or splinter hemorrhages.

Blood culture was positive for streptococcus, so he received penicillin (10 million units daily, I.V.) for 4 weeks. However, he continued to deteriorate, showing daily, progressive weakness, weight loss, dyspnea on exertion, and increasing signs of heart failure. After an echocardiogram and cardiac catheterization disclosed vegetations on the mitral valve, he was evaluated for possible valve replacement. The surgeon postponed this until heart failure and sepsis were relieved.

After 4 more weeks of treatment, Mr. Jarvis improved enough for mitral valve replacement. He had a successful porcine valve replacement and an uneventful postoperative recovery. He was discharged in good condition within 10 days of surgery.

Pericarditis
Pericarditis refers to inflammation of the pericardium. It can be acute or chronic constrictive. Constrictive pericarditis is due to chronic fibrotic disease of the pericardium, with or without calcification that impairs cardiac function. The most common form is fibrinous pericarditis.

Its predisposing factors include:
- infections (bacterial, viral, or fungal)
- systemic disease (rheumatoid arthritis, SLE [systemic lupus erythematosus], myocardial infarction, Dressler's syndrome)
- trauma to the chest or myocardium, and
- neoplasm (lymphomas).

In pericarditis, the inflammation commonly involves the lower portion of the parietal pericardium, an area that carries pain receptors. So, patients with pericarditis commonly complain of chest pain, especially...
- when they move the torso
- when they cough or take a deep breath
- when they are recumbent.

The rigid heart
One kind of acute pericarditis, called fibrinous or fibrotic, is commonly seen in rheumatic fever.

Such pain may be dull or sharp; precordial or substernal; and can radiate to the neck, trapezius, shoulder, and down the arms. Since this pain pattern is identical to that of myocardial infarction, careful assessment is crucial.

The most helpful clue? Pericardial pain usually changes with respiration and a change in body position. It diminishes when the patient sits up and leans forward (sitting up pulls the heart away from the diaphragmatic pleura of the lung).

Another classic sign is the pericardial friction rub. You can hear this sound by listening with your stethoscope over the patient's apical area. This sound is due to myocardial movement during atrial and ventricular systole, and ventricular diastole, which rubs the pericardium against the diaphragmatic pleura. Listen for an intermittent, transient, "to and fro" sound much like sand paper rubbing together.

Depending on the underlying cause, the patient may have associated symptoms: fever, dyspnea, chills, fatigue, or tachycardia. Therapy of pericarditis aims to remove the underlying cause and relieve symptoms. It usually includes: reassurance and support, bed rest, aspirin for fever and pain, and sometimes, steroids.

Patients may also develop pericardial effusion. If fluid accumulates rapidly between the pericardium and myocardium, cardiac compression, and tamponade could occur. Watch for decreased blood pressure, tachycardia, cool clammy skin, distended neck veins, elevated CVP, and pulsus paradoxus. If you see any of these symptoms, notify the doctor *immediately*. The patient will need pericardial tap, a pleuropericardial window or pericardiectomy to save his life. Serum lab studies may show an elevated leukocyte count, erythrocyte sedimentation rate (ESR) and SGOT. On EKG you may see low voltage of the P-QRS-T complex with S-T segment elevation and T wave inversion. However, these changes are nonspecific. More helpful are an echocardiogram to determine the amount of accumulating fluid, and X-rays to show an enlarged heart or pericardial effusion.

Rheumatic heart disease
Rheumatic heart disease denotes the cardiac involvement that follows rheumatic fever. Rheumatic fever, generally considered a childhood disease, has become much less common during the last 30 years because of the successful use of an-

tibiotics against streptococcal infections. But it does still occur. Rheumatic fever usually develops 2 to 3 weeks after acute pharyngitis due to hemolytic streptococci. It's an inflammatory disease caused by abnormal tissue reaction to an autoimmune mechanism. It affects various organs and tissues, and typically produces polyarthritis (usually of larger joints), subcutaneous nodules, and carditis (an acute inflammatory reaction of the heart muscle or pericardium). Roughly a third of the children with rheumatic fever have some signs of carditis during the acute stage. Such carditis can cause irreversible heart damage. Fortunately, in most children, it heals completely or leaves only insignificant scarring.

Clinical signs delayed

Remember, there's usually a long latent period between the first attack of rheumatic fever and a full-blown case of rheumatic heart disease. The patient usually lives a normal life without a hint of a problem. He may be told he has a murmur, but it causes him no difficulty. At age 30 or 40, cardiac symptoms may begin.

Mrs. Grant, a 32-year-old mother of two young children had rheumatic fever when she was 12. She had no symptoms after that until she was 31. Then she began to feel shortness of breath and slight chest discomfort after exercising, which she attributed to her age and lack of regular exercise. But when her symptoms recurred even with minimal exercise, she became worried and sought medical help. A thorough medical history and physical findings typical of valvular disease led to a diagnosis of rheumatic heart disease (see insert).

Rheumatic heart disease can mean extensive pathologic changes. During the acute inflammatory stages, rheumatic heart disease can affect all layers of the heart muscle producing: myocarditis (cardiac failure and hypertrophy may result); pericarditis (causing the surface of the heart to become reddened and rough, often with a fibrinous exudate); and endocarditis (involving the endocardium and valves, usually of the left side of the heart). The valve leaflets become edematous and inflamed, and vegetations appear along the closure line. The principal valvular sequelae of rheumatic heart disease are mitral and/or aortic regurgitation and mitral stenosis. Regurgitation results when inflammation and edema of the leaflets produce retraction of the leaflets and cusps; stenosis results

Signs and symptoms of valve disorders

MITRAL REGURGITATION
- Systolic murmur heard best at the apex and transmitted to the axilla, left sternal border, and base of the heart
- EKG — P wave abnormalities, atrial fibrillation, PACs
- Increasing fatigue and dyspnea.

MITRAL STENOSIS
- Diastolic murmur heard best over the apex, and transmitted to the axilla, epigastrium, left sternal border
- EKG — notched and peaked P waves, atrial fibrillation
- Increased fatigue with decreased exercise tolerance and dyspnea.

AORTIC REGURGITATION
- Decrescendo diastolic murmur of blowing quality heard best over left lower sternal border
- Loudest in aortic area and transmitted to the axilla and left sternal border
- EKG — left ventricular hypertrophy
- Dyspnea on exertion, bounding pulse with a rapid rise and fall; deMusset's sign, widened arterial pulse pressure.

when the leaflets become rigid with calcified adhesions of the cusps.

No laboratory test points specifically to rheumatic heart disease. However, some useful tests identify infective pathogens and measure inflammation via leukocyte count, sedimentation rate, and C-reactive protein. Echocardiograms identify the presence and severity of any valvular damage. Cardiac catheterization evaluates valvular disease and overall cardiac function in terms of left ventricular function and cardiac output.

Many patients with rheumatic heart disease never develop serious problems and lead completely normal lives. However, a certain percentage develop recurrent infections or signs of heart failure. So, medical management depends on: severity of valvular disease, the patient's symptoms, and any complications (SBE or heart failure). Treatment aims to relieve cardiac symptoms and sepsis (via antibiotics, low-sodium diet, diuretics, digitalis, beta-adrenergic blockers, and antiarrhythmic agents).

The same criteria determine surgical intervention. Is the patient symptomatic or septic? If so, how severely? Severe cases may require surgery, despite the risk, because of the danger of spontaneous rupture of the papillary muscles and the threat of embolism.

After valve surgery, patients need detailed information on diet, exercise, medications, and special precautions against infections. Make sure they understand their need for prophylactic antibiotic treatment during any dental work, or gastrointestinal or genitourinary procedures. Stress that they must remember to tell all dentists and doctors who treat them about their valve replacement.

Cardiomyopathy
Mysterious dysfunction

BY KATHLEEN A. DRACUP, RN, MN

TOM, A TALL, HANDSOME FRESHMAN from the local university really stood out among the much older patients in the Coronary Observation Unit. In his street clothes and tennis shoes, he looked and moved like the athlete he was. The only clue to his patient status was the Holter recording device strapped over his shoulder. What was an apparently healthy person doing in the COU? Three mornings ago, he had been jogging in the park. The next thing he remembered, he was lying on the ground looking into the faces of two paramedics and several fellow joggers. While running, he had suddenly collapsed. Luckily, the woman jogging behind him happened to be an anesthesiologist, who immediately started cardiopulmonary resuscitation. The paramedics, who arrived quickly, found him in ventricular fibrillation, which they successfully converted. He was awake and asking questions as they placed him on a stretcher and into the ambulance. Now, after 3 days of diagnostic tests, the doctors were telling him he had heart disease.

At the same time, Captain Morgan lay dying in the Coronary Care Unit nearby. A retired Air Force pilot, he had a long history of alcohol abuse. After multiple admissions during the past year for congestive heart failure, he was now unresponsive to treatment.

A third patient, Fernanda Moreno, a 38-year-old mother of a 6-week-old infant, was hospitalized in the CCU because she was having trouble breathing. She couldn't understand why she should still feel so weak when her recent labor and delivery had gone so well.

These three patients — seemingly so different — shared the same diagnosis: cardiomyopathy. The disparity in their ages and conditions truly reflects the nature of this disease. Actually, it's not one disease, but a group of diseases involving pathology of the heart muscle. It can affect young and old alike. Its cause is usually unknown and its prognosis, poor. Therefore, treatment is usually palliative, not curative. Patients with cardiomyopathy have to deal with a shortened life span, and with numerous changes in life-style (diet, medication, and exercise) demanded by medical treatment.

What is it?

Cardiomyopathy simply means heart (cardio) muscle (myo) disease (pathy). Other terms have also been used: myocardiopathy, idiopathic myocardial hypertrophy, idiopathic cardiomegaly, and primary myocardial disease, to name but a few. All of these terms describe a group of diseases which affect the myocardium without affecting other cardiovascular structures like the heart valves or the coronary arteries. Many cases of heart failure are now known to result from cardiomyopathy, rather than coronary artery obstruction or rheumatic myocarditis, or rheumatic valvular disease.

Much is still unknown about cardiomyopathy. But three of its features are almost universally accepted:

• The cause of the disease is unknown or unusual.

• It involves a disorder of the heart muscle, sometimes associated with endocardial and/or pericardial involvement.

• Cardiomegaly and heart failure predominate.

Cardiomyopathy may be primary (when the heart alone is involved) or secondary (when other organs are involved as well). Some examples of secondary cardiomyopathy: hemochromatosis (a metabolic disease characterized by excessive deposition of iron in the myocardium and other tissues); sarcoidosis; amyloidosis (which affects connective tissues); and certain neurological disorders (muscular dystrophy).

THREE KINDS OF CARDIOMYOPATHY

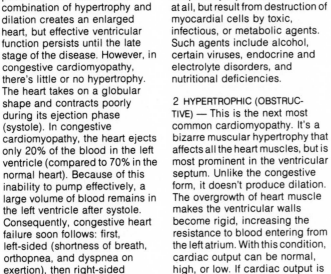

1 CONGESTIVE — Congestive cardiomyopathy is the most common form. It involves extensive damage to the myofibrils, interference with myocardial metabolism, and gross dilation of the heart. In other forms of heart disease that produce such dilation (such as aortic regurgitation), hypertrophy of the ventricular muscle keeps pace with the dilation. This combination of hypertrophy and dilation creates an enlarged heart, but effective ventricular function persists until the late stage of the disease. However, in congestive cardiomyopathy, there's little or no hypertrophy. The heart takes on a globular shape and contracts poorly during its ejection phase (systole). In congestive cardiomyopathy, the heart ejects only 20% of the blood in the left ventricle (compared to 70% in the normal heart). Because of this inability to pump effectively, a large volume of blood remains in the left ventricle after systole. Consequently, congestive heart failure soon follows: first, left-sided (shortness of breath, orthopnea, and dyspnea on exertion), then right-sided

(dependent edema, liver engorgement, and anasarca). Patients with congestive cardiomyopathy are usually hospitalized with heart failure, arrhythmias, and embolic phenomena. Typically, they have a large heart, gallop rhythms, and valvular insufficiency.

Many of the congestive cardiomyopathies are probably not primary myocardial disorders at all, but result from destruction of myocardial cells by toxic, infectious, or metabolic agents. Such agents include alcohol, certain viruses, endocrine and electrolyte disorders, and nutritional deficiencies.

2 HYPERTROPHIC (OBSTRUC-TIVE) — This is the next most common cardiomyopathy. It's a bizarre muscular hypertrophy that affects all the heart muscles, but is most prominent in the ventricular septum. Unlike the congestive form, it doesn't produce dilation. The overgrowth of heart muscle makes the ventricular walls become rigid, increasing the resistance to blood entering from the left atrium. With this condition, cardiac output can be normal, high, or low. If cardiac output is

high or normal, the patient may have no symptoms and may remain undiagnosed for years. Eventually, though, cardiac function deteriorates.

Roughly 80% of patients with hypertrophic cardiomyopathy have an obstruction in the left ventricular outflow tract. This obstruction results from the hypertrophied ventricular septum and the movement of the anterior mitral valve leaflet into the outflow tract during systole.

3 RESTRICTIVE — This rarest form may be easily misdiag-nosed as constrictive pericar-ditis. Restrictive cardiomyopathy involves an infiltration of the myocardium, endocardium, and subendocardium with fibroelastic tissue, similar to that in amyloid disease. This infiltra-tion makes the heart rigid, so it doesn't distend well in diastole or contract completely in systole. The end result is low cardiac output and eventually, the symp-toms of congestive failure (dys-pnea, orthopnea, edema, liver engorgement, and anasarca).

A fourth category, obliterative, is extremely rare in temperate climates.

Three forms of cardiomyopathy

Based on their physiological and clinical signs, heart muscle diseases can be divided into three major groups: congestive, hypertrophic, and restrictive (see page 127). A fourth category, obliterative, is extremely rare in temperate climates like the United States, and we will not discuss it here.

Many of the congestive cardiomyopathies are secondary disorders, the result of myocardial destruction by toxic, infectious, or metabolic agents. Occasionally, they may result from ischemic heart disease. Usually, however, patients with congestive cardiomyopathy have normal coronary arteries on arteriography.

One of the most commonly recognized toxic agents is *alcohol*, with or without malnutrition. Excessive ingestion of alcohol can produce severe congestive heart failure that tends to improve when the patient stops drinking, and recurs when he takes it up again. But not everyone who abuses alcohol develops alcoholic cardiomyopathy. Probably individual differences and susceptibilities, combined with other risk factors, explain this discrepancy.

Viruses may also produce congestive cardiomyopathy. Many investigators are studying a possible link between the viral infection of myocarditis and later development of congestive cardiomyopathy. The viruses currently implicated are coxsackievirus B, poliovirus, and influenza.

Metabolic cardiomyopathies follow *endocrine* and *electrolyte* disorders and nutritional deficiences. For example, hyperthyroidism, pheochromocytoma, beriberi (thiamine deficiency) and kwashiorkor (protein deficiency) have been associated with congestive cardiomyopathy.

One form of congestive cardiomyopathy does not fall neatly into any one of the above categories and is particularly poignant to deal with: postpartum or peripartum cardiomyopathy. It develops in some women in the last trimester or up to 5 months after delivery. Its cause is unknown, but is most common in multiparous women over 30. Treatment sometimes reverses this kind of cardiomegaly and congestive heart failure. If it does, these women can live on, and even have subsequent pregnancies without cardiac problems. But if cardiomegaly persists despite treatment, the prognosis is extremely poor.

In the United States, hypertrophic cardiomyopathy with

Key to the heart

Ambulatory electrocardiography, also known as Holter monitoring after Dr. Norman J. Holter who conceived and developed the process, enables a doctor to monitor as many as 100,000 cardiac cycles over a 24-hour period. The advantages of this method are many.

With very little equipment, the doctor can hook up a patient to one or more EKG leads. These record onto a portable cassette tape recorder (Figure 1) which the patient can wear easily.

The recorder should be connected to an EKG for test readings. After the hookup has been checked, the patient goes through a normal day (Figure 2) on the monitor. He is encouraged to try out those activities that bring on his symptoms, keeping a diary to record the exact times of symptoms, activities, and any drugs he takes so that their impact can be correlated with the EKG printouts. With the aid of a high-speed scanner (Figure 3), the doctor can review 24 hours of tape in 24 minutes, picking up important EKG changes.

Although not a substitute for CCU monitoring, the Holter monitor can catch a sporadic rhythm disturbance that an office or stress-test EKG might miss. It also saves the patient the time and expense of a hospital stay.

Holter monitoring has proved useful for patients recuperating from myocardial infarctions, those taking antiarrhythmic drugs, or those using pacemakers. It can catch rate, rhythm, and conduction abnormalities as well as cardiac responses to a normal environment. It is especially useful in diagnosing arrhythmias and the cause of CNS symptoms.

Ten common problems in cardiomyopathy patients
You can help a patient with cardiomyopathies by teaching him about his illness, what produces his symptoms, how to control them with medication, and how to pace his activities to avoid taxing his heart. His precarious condition may cause him severe psychiatric disturbances, so counsel him well and when necessary, refer him for psychosocial intervention.
   Expect to see:
1. Dyspnea secondary to heart failure
2. Syncope secondary to ventricular outflow tract obstruction (in IHSS)
3. Chest pain secondary to low cardiac output (in some patients only)
4. Fatigue secondary to inadequate cardiac output and/or heart failure
5. Anxiety (fear of sudden death)
6. Depression or hopelessness
7. Body image disturbance
8. Role disturbance
9. Forced dependency
10. Poor cooperation with prescribed treatment

obstruction is called *"idiopathic hypertrophic subaortic stenosis" (IHSS)*.

Patients with IHSS may have angina pectoris, palpitations or arrhythmias, dyspnea, syncope, and, rarely, congestive heart failure. They have a medium-pitched systolic ejection murmur heard along the left sternal border and at the apex. Their peripheral pulse has a characteristic double impulse (pulsus bisferiens).

Many patients with IHSS remain asymptomatic for a long time. The very first sign of the disease may be cardiac arrest, although the reason for susceptibility to fatal arrhythmias is not clear. As the disease progresses, the atria become dilated and atrial fibrillation common. In late stages, congestive heart failure occurs.

In restrictive cardiomyopathy, the heart becomes rigid so it doesn't adequately distend in diastole or contract in systole. Low cardiac output follows with its characteristic symptoms: easy fatigue, dyspnea on exertion, and symptoms of congestive heart failure. Fortunately, restrictive cardiomyopathy is extremely rare.

Diagnosis by exclusion
No special test can conclusively identify cardiomyopathy and this diagnosis is often made by excluding other possibilities. For example, electrocardiography and angiography can rule out ischemic heart disease in a patient with cardiomegaly, congestive heart failure, and vague chest pain. A chest X-ray reveals massive cardiomegaly that usually affects all four heart chambers, but no X-ray can specifically identify heart muscle disease. The characteristic EKG changes of biventricular hypertrophy and dilation can help identify cardiomyopathy. Cardiac catheterization and echocardiography are also helpful in diagnosing IHSS. Myocardial biopsy may support the diagnosis, but the test itself is risky and may yield a false negative unless the *entire* myocardium is diseased.

Most treatment palliative
When cardiomyopathy stems from some known cause such as alcohol or drugs, obviously the cause must be withdrawn. Of course, in alcoholic cardiomyopathy, removing the cause is not as easy as it sounds. But in most cases, the cause is unknown and, so, treatment is palliative rather than curative.

Overall, cardiomyopathy is a degenerative disease with a poor prognosis, but certain treatments do help, depending on the kind of cardiomyopathy.

In congestive cardiomyopathy, treatment aims to improve the heart's ability to function as a pump and to relieve symptoms of heart failure. Such treatment usually includes digitalis, diuretics, a low-sodium diet, and oxygen. It may also include steroids, prolonged bedrest, and pericardiotomy — which have given mixed results and need to be evaluated more fully.

In the last 5 years, vasodilators have been found effective in treating refractory heart failure in congestive cardiomyopathy. Their effectiveness has been attributed to the reduction of outflow (peripheral vascular) resistance. Possibly, vasodilators may also improve myocardial perfusion, which might be inadequate with dilated and hypertrophied muscle despite normal coronary arteries.

In the acutely ill patient, vasodilation can be achieved with intravenous infusion of sodium nitroprusside; later, it can be maintained with sublingual isosorbide dinitrate and oral phenoxybenzamine hydrochloride. These drugs relieve dyspnea and orthopnea by increasing cardiac output and decreasing pulmonary venous pressure. This treatment has given many former "cardiac cripples" new capabilities. Some patients with severe and incapacitating heart disease after treatment with vasodilators become relatively symptom-free and able to resume activities long since abandoned. This treatment is still only palliative, but it does control congestive heart failure in such patients.

In hypertrophic cardiomyopathies, treatment aims to relax the ventricle and relieve obstruction of the outflow tract. Since many of these patients are diagnosed in their teens or twenties (Tom, the young athlete, had typical IHSS), issues of exercise, diet modification, and life-long medication are crucial.

Surgical treatment has been tried with varying success. Ventricular myotomy (resection of the hypertrophied septum), and mitral valve replacement, alone or in conjunction with ventricular myotomy, have been tried. These techniques have noticeably eased outflow tract obstruction and have relieved symptoms, but surgical mortality is high (usually 10% to 20%). Because surgical intervention is only palliative and the prognosis so uncertain, such treatment is still considered experimental.

Medical treatment uses propranolol (Inderal), a beta adrenergic blocker), which effectively reduces angina, syncope,
dyspnea, and arrhythmias in patients with IHSS. In theory, it
should also inhibit tachycardia during exercise or stress, and
thus prevent sudden death. But available statistics do not yet
support this hope. Clearly, nurses need to cope with this
negative outlook in a practical way. For example, they should
persuade the patient's family to learn cardiopulmonary resuscitation. Warn patients who take Inderal against stopping it
abruptly. This can bring on a rebound of symptoms and sudden death.

In the end stage of the disease, atrial fibrillation usually
develops. Digitalis and/or cardioversion can usually successfully convert the rhythm. Since there's a great risk of systemic
embolism, the patient needs anticoagulants as long as he's in
atrial fibrillation. Keep in mind that *while vasodilators and
inotropic agents are a great help to patients with congestive
cardiomyopthy, the decrease in outflow resistance achieved
by arterial vasodilation and venous pooling increases obstruction in the outflow tract of the patient with IHSS.* Remember
this, because some of the patients develop chest pain. *You
might be tempted to use standing orders for nitroglycerin. But
if you do, such a patient's obstruction will worsen and may
lead to syncope and sudden death.*

In restrictive cardiomyopathies, treatment includes digitalis, diuretics, and a low-sodium diet (to improve contractility
of the heart and reduce resistance during systole and diastole);
and oral vasodilators (isosorbide dinitrate and phenoxybenzamine) to treat the intractable congestive failure. Monitor
these patients carefully (especially blood pressure and urine
output), when treatment with vasodilators begins. If acutely
ill, they may need hemodynamic monitoring with the Swan-
Ganz pulmonary catheter.

Pulmonary Embolism
Hazard of immobilization

BY M. SANDY WYPER, RN, MSN

PULMONARY EMBOLISM strikes young and old, men and women, in the hospital and on the street. In hospitalized patients, it is the most common pulmonary complication. To cope with this exceedingly common problem, you need to know what conditions make pulmonary embolism a likely complication...How to care for patients with an embolism.... Most important, you need to know what nursing measures can help prevent it.

Who gets it?
It's especially likely among immobilized patients; those recovering from surgery; patients with myocardial infarction, cerebrovascular accidents, congestive heart failure, fractures, and burns; and elderly patients with debilitating diseases. Mr. Andrews, a 69-year-old laborer, was recovering from a medullary stroke in the rehabilitation unit of a general hospital. Twenty days after admission, he awoke from an afternoon nap complaining of dyspnea and a dull, diffuse chest pain. His respirations were rapid but he was not cyanotic. His systolic blood pressure had fallen to 95 mm Hg. His nurse called a doctor, elevated the head of the bed 45 degrees, and started

What is pulmonary embolism?

It is any obstruction of the pulmonary vascular bed. Typically, a dislodged thrombus causes such obstruction, but it can be caused by any foreign substance.

Thromboembolism: Of the pulmonary emboli caused by a dislodged thrombi, 75% originate in the peripheral venous system (almost half of these in the deep veins of the lower extremities); 10% in pelvic veins; and 10% in the right heart chamber.

A *fat embolism* commonly follows fracture of long bones and other trauma such as closed-chest massage, burns, nephritis, infections, and liver disease (including that induced by alcoholism).

An *air embolism* may be caused by improper technique in administering intravenous infusions or any procedure in which air is injected into a body cavity.

Amniotic fluid emboli may follow complications of pregnancy including intrauterine fetal death and placenta previa. The amniotic fluid itself predisposes to deposition of fibrin throughout the venous system. Moreover, the solid contents of the fluid such as lipids and lanugo hair may embolize.

Tumor emboli, which may embolize from either primary or metastatic sites, probably occur more frequently than is generally thought.

oxygen by mask to relieve his dyspnea. She also started an I.V. to avoid difficulty later, if his blood pressure continued to drop.

Physical examination showed that the chest was clear. But an EKG showed a rapid, regular heart rate of 150 beats per minute. The arrhythmia converted to normal sinus rhythm after 3 mg of I.V. propranolol (Inderal) and the application of carotid sinus pressure. This response to treatment made paroxysmal atrial tachycardia the most likely diagnosis. The dyspnea and pain subsided within a few minutes. The only other notable finding was mild tenderness in the calf which the patient said had been present for several months.

The attending staff considered several possible causes. A simple bout of arrhythmia that decreased cardiac output sufficiently to cause angina? A myocardial infarction? Both were possible, but pulmonary embolism was most likely in view of the calf pain, and the patient's long immobilization.

Mr. Andrews was transferred to an acute medical unit for further evaluation. At the time of the transfer, his blood gases showed a low PO_2 (80) and a low PCO_2 (33). Mr. Andrews had a history of GI bleeding, so anticoagulation was inadvisable without a certain diagnosis of pulmonary embolism. A lung scan showed a perfusion defect in the right lower lung field which did not correlate with any abnormality on X-ray. This confirmed pulmonary embolism and anticoagulant treatment began.

Mr. Andrews' pulmonary embolism was decidedly atypical in that it was immediately suspected and quickly confirmed. Generally, recognizing a pulmonary embolus is much more difficult. Fewer than half of pulmonary emboli are detected while the patient is alive! Consequently, prevention is doubly important. But to prevent most emboli, you must prevent the formation of thrombi.

What causes thrombi?

Three conditions predispose to thrombus formation: hypercoagulability of the blood; alterations in the integrity of blood vessel walls; and venous stasis (see page 160). Obviously preventing thrombus formation requires prevention of these three conditions. Unfortunately, little can be done to prevent hypercoagulability except for the kind that follows abrupt discontinuation of anticoagulants. Prevent this by teaching patients who take anticoagulants not to discontinue them without a doctor's supervision.

You can do several things to minimize damage to vessel walls. First, of course, avoid venipuncture trauma by placing intravenous needles carefully. Also, avoid placing I.V.s in leg and pelvic veins, which have the greatest tendency to thrombus formation. Also minimize vessel wall damage associated with chronic conditions by frequently changing the patient's body position. Such changes shift pressure points and stimulate neural reflexes that help prevent venous distention and thus prevent pooling in dependent areas. Encourage patients who can move without help to do so often. Be sure they understand the dangers of remaining in one position too long or of allowing prolonged pressure on one area (as happens when sitting with legs crossed). Healthy people *automatically* change their body position at least every 30 minutes. So remember to help immobilized patients frequently. Never make them wait for the minimum q2h turnings we often find on nursing care plans.

Venous stasis causes clots and also extends existing clots. Thus, it can complicate all other thrombus-associated conditions. Venous stasis is sometimes linked to obesity, congestive heart failure, and certain arrhythmias. But its most important predisposing factor is long-term immobility. In immobile patients like Mr. Andrews, bedrest decreases blood flow by approximately 50% because of the loss of muscle tone, which normally assists in pushing blood back to the heart. Immobilization also causes generalized vasodilation (from increased parasympathetic nervous system activity) and this, in turn, promotes pooling in dependent areas. Much can be done to prevent this major cause of thrombus formation. And you're usually the one who can do it. How to prevent thrombus formation?

Encourage ambulation
The trend toward early ambulation after surgery and to a limited extent after myocardial infarction has prevented venous stasis in many patients. To encourage early ambulation, you must explain the need for it to get the patient's cooperation. Encourage self-care as prescribed, while keeping track of its effect on the patient's cardiovascular status and well-being. Continue to monitor the heart rate and watch for arrhythmia.

Bend and stretch
A bedridden patient needs exercise to prevent venous stasis. If he can't move, help him with passive exercises.
  1. Place one hand under the patient's knee and your other hand on his heel.
  2. Lift his leg. Bend it at the knee.

Don't allow the patient to exercise to the point of exhaustion. (It's worth remembering that patients find using a bedside commode much less exhausting than using a bedpan.)

Encourage exercise

Every nurse can glibly recite the maneuvers that supposedly prevent venous stasis in the bedridden patient. But not nearly so many practice these maneuvers with the required zeal. Admittedly, teaching a reluctant patient to exercise properly can be frustrating. And many nurses have been discouraged by statements that the standard preventive measures do not really decrease thrombus formation. If you have been discouraged by such statements, you should know that a United States Public Health Service report cites disability from immobilization as one of the top ten preventable health problems. This report also suggests that these disabilities could probably be reduced by 50 to 75%. That's strong support for vigorous nursing measures.

What nursing measures may be most effective? Because over 75% of embolized thrombi originate in the main venous channels of the lower leg, most preventive measures emphasize positioning and exercising of the legs, elastic stockings or bandages, and deep-breathing exercises.

Prevent embolization

Once you detect thrombus or, in some cases, simply because the risk of a thrombus is great, take precautions to keep the thrombus from breaking loose. You may be able to give anticoagulants to prevent further clot formation and apply heat locally to reduce pain and inflammation. Avoid trauma to the threatened area and maintain a steady flow-rate. To maintain a steady flow-rate, teach patients to avoid sudden exertion or any sudden movements of the legs and, particularly, to avoid holding their breath and bearing down in the Valsalva maneuver. They are especially likely to do this when having a bowel movement or when turning in bed. As you know, the Valsalva maneuver may cause reflex slowing of heart rate or temporary heart block. The great danger to a patient with a thrombus is that such straining also greatly increases intrathoracic pressure, which reduces venous return. When the patient stops straining, release of pressure allows a sudden surge of venous flow, which may dislodge a thrombus.

How to recognize pulmonary embolism?

The signs, symptoms, and laboratory findings depend on the size and location of the embolus.

Large embolus: Acute cor pulmonale. Acute cor pulmonale results from an embolus large enough to occlude the pulmonary artery or one of its major branches. It usually produces a clear-cut clinical picture: pulmonary hypertension coupled with decreased venous return to the left heart and thus impaired systemic circulation. At the same time, increased pressure proximal to the obstruction increases venous pressure producing neck-vein distention, increased CVP readings, and abdominal tenderness due to liver congestion. An EKG tracing taken soon after onset of symptoms may show changes characteristic of right heart strain. Atrial arrhythmias may follow distention of the right atrium; murmurs of tricuspid or pulmonic insufficiency may follow increased right ventricular volume.

The obstruction to circulation through the lungs produces profound hemodynamic effects. In addition to the inevitable hypoxia, decreased venous return to the left heart causes decreased ventricular filling. Hypotension develops, and the patient becomes pale, tachycardic, and apprehensive. Decreased coronary and cerebral perfusion appear as anginal pain and mental confusion. This clinical picture rarely calls for further diagnostic tests. (An exception: Pulmonary angiograms are needed before embolectomy.)

Medium embolus: Infarction. Pulmonary infarction (necrosis of lung tissue) may occur when an embolus occludes a medium sized artery and decreases circulation to the surrounding pulmonary parenchyma by the bronchial arteries. Systemic hypotension or pulmonary venous hypertension compromises bronchial circulation and is most likely in patients with infected, congested, or hypoventilated lungs. Pulmonary infarction is not usually fatal, and often facilitates the diagnosis of pulmonary embolism. Still, its symptoms and physical findings vary from patient to patient, so you must watch for its most prevalent findings to recognize it.

Small and medium emboli: Varying symptoms. Some small emboli produce no symptoms at all. Others can mimic a myocardial infarction, dissecting aortic aneurysm, pericarditis, congestive heart failure, pneumonia, bronchitis, and simple episodes of arrhythmias.

What are its usual symptoms? Most patients develop dyspnea and a cough. Many patients complain of feelings of apprehension

3. Move his leg slowly back toward his head as far as it will go without hurting him.
4. Straighten his knee by lifting the foot upward. Lower his leg to the starting position and repeat the exercise.

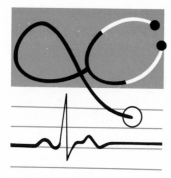

Diagnostic profile

LAB TESTS
WBC — If infarction is present, may be normal or elevated but is usually less than 15,000, with little or no increase in differential count. This helps rule out acute pneumonia in which the WBC often exceeds 15,000.
PO_2 — decreased; not above 90 and often below 80 mm Hg.
PCO_2 — below the normal (34 to 46 mm Hg).

ELECTROCARDIOGRAM
Circulatory obstruction *may* cause:
• right axis deviation
• right bundle branch block pattern in V_1
• sinus tachycardia
• tall peaked P waves (P pulmonale)
• shifts in S-T segment and T wave directions
• sudden onset of atrial flutter, atrial fibrillation, or other supraventricular tachycardias.

CHEST X-RAY
You may see a diaphragm elevation; pleural fluid on the affected side; and prominence of a pulmonary artery. A triangular shadow, indicating necrosis, may appear in pulmonary infarction patients. It's diagnostic.

or impending disaster. More than half have pain, usually in the chest but occasionally in the abdomen or flank. The character of the pain ranges from pleuritic to a close mimic of angina. Relatively few have hemoptysis (only 40% of emboli with infarctions). Cyanosis is rare.

Physical findings are even less specific. The combination of unexplained tachycardia, tachypnea, and fever is generally considered most characteristic of pulmonary embolism, but these same findings preexist in many patients with other pulmonary or cardiac diseases. However, four findings occur regularly in at least half of all patients: 1) an increased intensity of the pulmonic component of the second heart sound due to pulmonary hypertension (in about 80%); 2) tachypnea — more than 20 respirations per minute (in 75%); 3) pulmonary rales (in 70%); and 4) tachycardia (in 65%). Less often, patients may have an abnormal third heart sound (S_3 gallop), phlebitis, fever, and a pleural friction rub (fever and pleural friction rub are more typical of infarction than of simple embolus).

Because clinical findings are so inconclusive, the following diagnostic tests are generally ordered to confirm pulmonary embolism:

• Lab studies, as shown on the left, usually include white blood count, erythrocyte sedimentation rate, serum enzymes, and arterial blood gases.

• A chest X-ray rules out other pulmonary pathology.

• A lung scan is one of the most useful confirming procedures (see page 139).

• An EKG may distinguish between acute myocardial infarction and pulmonary embolism.

• Pulmonary angiography is the most definitive test. Through a dye-injection technique, angiography pinpoints the exact location of an embolus in the pulmonary arterial tree.

Treatment two-fold

The treatment of acute pulmonary embolism requires support of vital functions and prevention of further emboli. Death, when it occurs, is due to circulatory failure, and 3 out of 4 such deaths occur within a few hours. In patients who survive, circulation begins to seep past the clot as pressure builds up next to it. Improvement thereafter is usually rapid.

Treatment measures include:

• *Bedrest* is necessary to prevent further embolization, but the

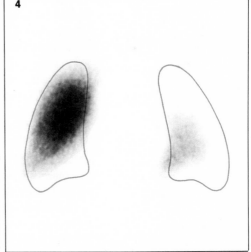

What lung scans show

Lung scans show pulmonary blood flow. Emboli too small to be picked up by angiogram can be seen on a lung scan. Blood perfusion is shown by the dark areas. Figure 1 shows a normal lung scan.

Often ordered in conjunction with the scan is an equilibrium test. For this test, the patient inhales an inert gas, such as xenon, along with oxygen for 30 seconds. The scan which photographs xenon then shows lung ventilation. Figure 2 shows a normal equilibrium.

To assess the total lung field, scans are taken from two different views. Figure 3 shows an anterior view and Figure 4 shows a posterior view. In both cases you can see that the right apical segment is incompletely perfused due to a pulmonary embolus.

Hints on heparin

Heparin is commonly administered by I.V. intermittent bolus injection. Since it has a short half-life — about 60 minutes — never give bolus doses more often than every 4 hours. To check effectiveness, draw blood for the partial thromboplastin time (PTT) test half an hour before the next heparin dose is due. Adjust dosage to achieve a therapeutic level that is 2½ times the normal control, which is 35 to 45 seconds.

Continuous infusion produces less bleeding (an incidence 8 to 10 times lower) than bolus injections, but it needs close monitoring. Use an I.V. pump or controller to prevent inadvertent overdose by too fast an infusion. Or, use a 100-ml burette chamber and fill it hourly.

Don't delay giving heparin because blood isn't drawn in time or you haven't received lab results. Notify the doctor that heparin is due. If you can't reach him in 5 minutes, give the heparin on schedule and then try to reach the doctor and inform him why the blood wasn't drawn. Withhold heparin only if the patient has nosebleeds, ecchymoses, bloody urine, or other side effects. In that case, notify the doctor immediately.

Don't be alarmed if the doctor prescribes a high dose of heparin. Because pulmonary embolism decreases heparin's half-life, patients with this condition require a higher-than-normal initial dose.

Of course, policies vary from institution to institution, so make sure you know your own hospital's rules about heparin before using it.

nurse must be prepared to combat all the additional hazards of immobility.

- *Oxygen* is given either by mask or by cannula.
- *Vasopressors* may be used for severe circulatory failure.
- *Heparin* is given in an initial I.V. injection of 10,000 to 15,000 units. (Subcutaneous administration is rarely used because of uneven absorption with this route.) Subsequent dosage is regulated to achieve a clotting time of 25 to 35 minutes. Oral anticoagulation may be started at the same time or delayed for a few days. Most patients can begin oral use after 4 to 7 days of heparin.
- *Narcotics* to relieve pain and apprehension.
- *Digitalization* may begin (although at less than full digitalizing dose because myocardial ischemia can result from poor coronary artery perfusion).
- *Intravenous fluids* may be given to combat shock. If so, monitor central venous pressure.
- *Thrombolytic agents* such as urokinase (Abbokinase) and streptokinase (Streptase) may be used to dissolve the embolus and the original thrombus.
- *Embolectomy* is considered only in patients who have profound circulatory failure or who cannot be anticoagulated. Pulmonary angiography must be done first to exactly locate the obstruction. Embolectomy sometimes fails because emboli are too small to be easily removed. Also, mortality is high, largely because of the patient's poor condition before surgery.
- *Calm reassurance* may be your most important contribution. The frightening onset of symptoms and the bustling activity they elicit from the health-care team are sure to produce extreme anxiety in the patient and his family. You can help a great deal by keeping the aura of crisis to a minimum.

Once a patient has had a pulmonary embolus, he forever has a greater risk of re-embolization. Your greatest challenge lies in helping such patients accept a lifetime program of thrombus prevention — something they find difficult when they feel well. It's your job to stress the need for continuing medical surveillance. Teach patients "at risk" to continue their anticoagulation and monitor their daily activities to prevent venous stasis. Some patients cooperate poorly with any drug regimen. Still others develop recurrent emboli despite vigorous anticoagulation treatment. Such patients may eventually need surgical interruption of the inferior vena cava.

14

Pacemakers
Help for the faltering heart

BY MINNIE BOWEN ROSE, RN, BSN, MEd

MR. MACKENZIE WAS WORKING as a night clerk in a small hotel when he fell and couldn't get up. An ambulance brought him to the emergency room where he seemed weak and slightly confused. His heart rate was 48; his blood pressure, 169/80. He didn't seem to be in acute distress. But when an EKG strip showed third-degree atrioventricular block, Mr. Mackenzie became a candidate for artificial pacing of his heart, and was admitted for cardiac evaluation.

The number of patients with pacemakers is growing every year and, chances are, you'll work with someone like Mr. Mackenzie sooner or later. Do you know all you really should about pacemakers? How to detect failure in their mechanism? How to answer patients' questions about them and properly prepare them to live with a pacemaker? If not, you may benefit from reading this chapter.

Pacemakers are increasingly being implanted temporarily in hospitalized patients — those with transient blockage of conductive pathways from edema, ischemia from coronary artery disease or following heart surgery, or myocardial infarction. For example, after heart surgery, while the chest is still open, surgeons routinely implant pacing electrodes on the epicar-

Patients for pacing

In the early days of pacemaking, the sole indication was complete atrioventricular block leading to Stokes-Adams attacks. Nowadays, doctors implant pacemakers for many conduction defects, ranging from complete to partial and/or intermittent AV block. Accepted indications include:

• complete AV block lasting 1 to 3 weeks or more following acute myocardial infarction

• complete AV block associated with congestive heart failure or cerebral or renal insufficiency that improves with temporary pacing

• persistent AV block following cardiac surgery

• need for prophylaxis following cardiac surgery

• incomplete AV block (Mobitz Type II or advanced second-degree block)

• symptomatic bilateral bundle branch block

• symptomatic sinus bradycardia, with or without AV block

• sinus arrest or sinoatrial block

• sick sinus syndrome

• trifascicular block

• atrial tachycardia

• need for improved cardiac output.

dium. They extend them through the chest incision and connect them to an external pacing battery box. The pacemaker is then a ready backup to be used as needed within the next few days: to control any arrhythmias that may develop after surgery; to increase the heart rate; or to improve cardiac output (if low output is due to brady- or tachyarrhythmias).

Artificial electric pacing almost always begins with a temporary transvenous pacemaker. Most implants are made through the subclavian, antecubital, external jugular, or femoral vein. A temporary pacemaker is relatively simple for the trained doctor to insert. It needs neither general anesthesia nor thoracotomy, but only a venous cutdown or percutaneous placement under local anesthesia. Its batteries are easy to replace, and the device can easily be removed when pacing is no longer needed.

Of course, temporary pacemakers have some obvious disadvantages: A disoriented patient can pull the catheter; electrodes may break, be dislodged, or perforate the ventricular wall; or the site of insertion can become infected. Then, too, the patient's constant awareness of being hooked up to external lifesaving equipment may cause him marked anxiety.

Permanent pacing

When a patient has irreversible cardiac damage with a complete block in the conduction system of the heart, he needs a permanent pacemaker. It, too, can be inserted intravenously. The difference between this and the temporary pacer is that its generator gets permanently implanted within the subcutaneous tissue of the patient's chest or abdomen.

Less often, the permanent electrodes get implanted transthoracically. The surgeon opens the chest anteriorly and sutures the electrodes into the epicardial surface of the ventricle. Then he threads the wires through a subcutaneous tunnel to the battery box, and sets them under the chest or abdominal skin. The chief drawback in this method: The patient must endure a major operation and the usual postoperative course of a thoracotomy. Problems with permanent pacemakers are relatively few. But infection at the implantation site is possible; any malfunction requires another surgical procedure.

Prepare patients for pacing

Pacemakers have saved countless lives. Yet, beyond a doubt,

the patient who has one is acutely aware of his dependence on this artificial heartbeat. Anything you can do to prepare him for it, help him get used to it, and teach him to live with it at home is a valuable service indeed. You'll usually be working with someone elderly; 70% of pacemaker patients are over 60. But some are young people, including infants born with a heart block. Men outnumber women 2 to 1.

Because the patient will surely forget some of what the surgeon tells him before the operation, it's a good idea for you to be there for the explanation. You can help him absorb it later. For example, you can tell him that the actual insertion of the device will be done through a small incision and under local anesthesia.

If he's getting a permanent pacemaker, show him a model of it and let him handle it. To minimize complications, emphasize the need for him to return to activity. According to his response to this advice, help him determine goals. Above all, help him understand that a pacemaker can return him to an active life his own heartbeat can no longer support. Try to explain all this to his family or closest relative, too, if possible while family and patient are together. Naturally they'll be worried. Remember to warn them kindly that getting through the operation successfully does not automatically guarantee recovery without complications.

It seems easier to prepare a patient for temporary pacing than for permanent pacing. Nonetheless, the short-term patient is often more apprehensive because the whole situation is so new to him. With patience and understanding, you can help him over this critical stage. You can help reduce the physiologic strain his emotions are adding to an already overtaxed heart.

After implantation

The patient will probably need bedrest for the rest of the day, and maybe for 48 hours. But after that, he should get up and walk around as soon as possible.

Resume your monitoring and run an EKG strip immediately for analysis of the pacemaker function. Check the incision site for bleeding, redness, warmth of the incision site, swelling, or pain. Expect some normal bloody drainage, but keep the skin as clean and dry as possible. Take vital signs as ordered and check for fever. Check the prescribed setting of the pacemaker, and record it in your notes. If things are going well, revise your nursing care plan to include patient-teaching requirements — especially if the patient has, or is going to have, a permanent device.

Keep the cardiac monitor going for about 24 hours to be sure the pacemaker is functioning properly and the electrodes haven't dislodged. Explain the importance of his continued monitoring meantime, and tell why you must watch his vital functions closely. Urge him to report any symptoms: faintness, hiccups, or pain. Patients usually have some pain at the operative site and need an analgesic. However, report persistent or increasing pain to the doctor. Make nursing observations frequently, and keep checking vital signs.

Watch for complications
Complications that may follow thoracic installation of the pacemaker? They primarily result from the chest surgery itself: pneumonia, atelectasis, embolism, or the like. So, the patient will need deep-breathing, intermittent positive-pressure breathing, coughing, and regular turning from side to side. These measures will help loosen bronchial secretions and keep lungs well expanded.

Certain complications may follow implantation of any kind of pacemaker. You need to recognize them promptly.

• *An electrode may break (infrequently) or be dislodged.* Then the QRS complex, which signifies contraction of the ventricles, will change contour on the cardiac monitor. The heart rate itself will noticeably slow down if pacing fails. When this happens the electrode must be repaired, replaced, or repositioned.

• *An electrode may perforate the ventricle wall.* Watch for hiccups, a sign of spasm of the upper-abdominal or lower-chest muscles stimulated by a stray electrode; you may save the patient's life. Also be alert for cardiac tamponade, in which blood in the pericardium compresses the heart. The signs of tamponade are low blood pressure, increased venous pressure, distended neck veins, increased pulse rate, decreased urinary output, cyanosis, and restlessness. If you suspect cardiac tamponade or stray electrode, notify the doctor at once: Immediate surgery is needed.

• *The pacemaker may malfunction; the heart may resist.* For the first 2 or 3 days after implantation, the heart is highly

Keeping pace

Temporary transvenous pacemakers (as shown in the figure on the left) are inserted via the groin or a cutdown in the arm. With a fluoroscope the doctor threads the catheter through a vein to the right ventricle. The most common site for permanent pacemaker implantation (as shown in the figure on the right) is a pocket the doctor forms in the right anterior chest. From here he threads the catheter through a vein — most commonly the right cephalic — into the right ventricle.

KINDS OF PACEMAKERS

FIXED-RATE ASYNCHRONOUS
—contain no sensing mechanism;
—fire continuously without regard to the patient's own rhythm;
—located in either the atrium or the ventricle.

DEMAND PACEMAKERS — all have both sensing and pre-set stimulating mechanisms.

R-wave inhibited: Can be temporary (Figure 1) or permanent (Figure 2). In the presence of the patient's own QRS complex, the pacemaker will not fire; the spike is inhibited. This is a true demand pacemaker, firing only when needed. It's the most common unit used.

• *R-triggered synchronized:* This pacemaker senses the patient's QRS complex and fires in the middle of it. Consequently,

it's not a true demand pacemaker, because it doesn't fire only when needed. Now, what happens if the QRS complex is delayed? Remember, all sensing pacemakers have preset intervals, so they will fire when no QRS complex is sensed. Disadvantage: Although the pacemaker's spike indicates a functional sensing mechanism, it does change the shape of the QRS complex. This may interfere with accurate interpretation of the patient's EKG.

• Bifocal sequential, QRS inhibited: This pacemaker has two electrodes, located in the atrium and in the ventricle, and contains both a sensing and stimulating mechanism. The sensing mechanism causes two spikes to fire in sequence, one before the P wave and one before the QRS

complex: A ventricular contraction will follow an atrial contraction. The P spike and the QRS spike represent the P-R interval.
—This pacemaker is also R-wave inhibited and fires only when needed.
—It can pace the atrium alone, pace the atrium and the ventricle in sequence, or remain dormant.
—It automatically adapts to the patient's needs and preserves the natural sequence of depolarization. Thus it combines the advantages of atrial, sequential, and demand pacing.
—It improves cardiac output by increasing heart rate as well as atrial contribution. It's also used for patients with sick sinus syndrome.

QUESTIONS PACEMAKER PATIENTS ASK

What am I allowed to do now that I have a pacemaker?
Generally, anything you enjoyed before. You can even play sports, as soon as the doctor gives you permission. He'll probably have you begin by walking and then gradually increase your activity. You should even be able to swim. The only athletic restriction you must observe is to avoid body contact sports, such as football.

As to sex, you can return to whatever degree of activity you want and can tolerate.

Can I return to work?
Yes, whenever the doctor says you may. Talk over your work with him to review what it entails. If you're a telephone linesman, you may have to switch to less strenuous work in a repair shop or in the office. If you're a banker or an accountant, you should be able to resume your duties. Jobs that involve working near equipment that can disrupt pacing (such as high tension wires and electrical generators) are unsuitable.

What daily medical care must I practice? Do I have to check my pulse often?
Yes, at least once a day for 60 seconds. The nurse will show you how, and what variations mean. Have a family member learn along with you. Keep a daily record of your pulse rate to bring to your next checkup. If your pulse rate drops below that set by the pacemaker, notify your doctor.

The nurse will explain your medications to you, and any precautions they require. Follow your doctor's orders about diet.

Take your medications faithfully as prescribed. Don't skip doses or vary the times you take them. Keep a record of what you take and when you take it, and bring

this along with your pulse record to your next checkup.

Can water hurt my pacemaker?
Don't wet the incision site until after the doctor removes the sutures and the site has completely healed. After that, however, any amount of water won't hurt.

How do I care for my incision?
Be careful to keep it clean and dry until it heals. Otherwise, you need no other special care.

Don't wear clothing that rubs or presses against the slight bump on your chest over the pacemaker unit. For example, a woman with a chest implant shouldn't wear tight bras. Similarly, patients with abdominal implants should avoid tight girdles.

If you notice redness, discharge, or pain over the implant, report it to your doctor.

What else should I watch for?
Call the doctor to report any dizziness, vertigo, shortness of breath, unwarranted fatigue, prolonged hiccups, nausea, vomiting, or diarrhea, or a very fast or very slow heart rate.

Can I travel?
Yes, you can resume driving a car after about a month, but avoid lengthy travel of any kind for at least 3 months after implant and then again during the later stages of battery life. Tell your doctor of your plans before you travel, and carry a list of doctors and hospitals in the appropriate locales to use in case of an emergency.

Pacemaker patients should always carry an ID card that gives a medical summary, the kind of pacemaker they have, its rate, and their doctor's name, address, and telephone number.

May I fly in a plane?
Yes, but if you must pass through an airport metal detector, alert the authorities that you have a pacemaker since the metal in it may set off an alarm.

Can electrical equipment harm me?
In general, no. Household appliances, if properly grounded, can't disrupt your pacemaker. But avoid using an electric shaver directly over the implanted unit. Also avoid standing or leaning over electric motors or gasoline engines. They can cause palpitations or an irregular heart rate and make you feel faint. But this will stop if you leave the area. For the same reasons, stay well out of the high-voltage electric fields that emanate from overhead utility transmission lines.

If you're having your teeth fixed or must have surgery, tell your dentist or surgeon that you have a pacemaker. You might need to take a prophylactic antibiotic to prevent any bloodborne infections. Consult your cardiologist before undergoing any medical procedure that involves electricity.

How long will my pacemaker last?
Some last at least 18 to 24 months, and most last longer.

What happens if it stops working?
Don't lose sleep over this! Your pacemaker clinic will replace the unit before it stops. Changing batteries involves only a simple procedure. But if the pacemaker does stop, the heart will slow to its former rate.

Visit your doctor for regular checkups, not because your pacemaker may fail but because your needs may change and your pacemaker may need resetting.

Pacemaker tips

- Explain to the patient why the procedure is necessary and how it will be performed.
- Show the patient a pacemaker; explain how it works.
- Watch him carefully after insertion to verify that the pacemaker is functioning properly and effectively.
- Watch for loss of capture, competition, signs of perforation, thrombophlebitis, or skin infection.
- Tell the patient and his family at what rate his pacemaker is set.

TEMPORARY PACEMAKER

- After the electrode has been introduced, gradually turn the energy control dial clockwise until you note a QRS complex with each stimulus. This is the patient's threshold level (usually about 1.5 milliamperes). As a safety precaution, this number is usually doubled to assure continued pacing.
- If loss of capture occurs:

(continued, opposite page)

sensitive to the electrode within it. Especially during that time, look for any disturbance in cardiac rhythm, such as PVCs and runs of ventricular tachycardia; signs of pacemaker failure, changing of rate, failure to capture, and return of symptoms such as syncope; or need to adjust the pacing rate. In some hospitals, you may be allowed to adjust the rate and sensitivity on an external power generator as necessary. In others, you can only monitor and report changes.

If the monitor shows premature ventricular extrasystoles or other ectopic activity, the patient may need immediate treatment with: antiarrhythmic drugs, restoration of normal potassium balance, or an increase in the pacing rate.

- *Watch for infection.* Contamination of the equipment or wound during the procedure or afterward can produce thrombophlebitis, septicemia, or endocarditis. You can help avoid these by using a rigorously aseptic technique in preparing the site, and later by watching the patient for any signs of infection.
- *Keep the extremity mobile.* When a temporary pacemaker is inserted in the antecubital vein, the patient's elbow must, of course, be immobilized to protect the site of insertion. Nevertheless, the patient needs to wiggle his fingers freely. He needs some range-of-motion exercises for his shoulder to avoid stiffness. Encourage every patient with permanent pacemakers in the upper-outer chest wall to exercise the arm on that side before and after the implantation. However, such exercises, any over-the-head motion of the arms, or any turning on the side should not begin for 24 to 72 hours after implantation (to avoid dislodgement of the catheter tip).

Troubleshooting the pacemaker

Suspect malfunction when you see symptoms of heart block return — such as syncope, slow pulse, and convulsions. Also suspect it when you see premature beats or changes in rhythm.

In many hospitals, an EKG technician will check a patient's temporary pacemaker daily. But you can check its function yourself. It's simple. With a stethoscope, listen to the patient's apical pulse and watch the sense-pace dial (on a temporary pulse generator). Use the apical pulse because the radial pulse is far enough away from the heart that the lag time between heartbeat and pulse is too great, particularly at faster rates. Whenever you suspect pacemaker malfunction, check the patient's pulse rate, blood pressure, level of consciousness, and respiratory status. If the apical rate has dropped too much, perfusion may be inadequate, and the patient may be at risk for cardiac arrest.

Firing: If the sense-pace dial on a temporary pacemaker generator shows the pacer has fired, and a split-second later you hear the pulse, you know the pacer is firing and capturing properly. If the sense-pace is *not* registering, you know the pacemaker has stopped firing. The usual cause: Someone inadvertently turned off the power switch. Other causes are malfunctioning electronic circuitry and dead batteries in the pulse generator. So, make sure the power switch is on, check all connections, and change the battery in the pulse generator. If firing doesn't resume, replace the pulse generator.

Capturing: If the sense-pace dial shows firing, but you hear no corresponding apical pulse, you know the pacemaker is not capturing. Suspect loss of capture when the patient's heart rate is less than the rate set on the pulse generator. Loss of capture usually results from displacement of the catheter tip. The tip is often wedged behind the trabeculae in the wall near the apex of the right ventricle. The tip may dislodge and float freely in the right ventricle, may advance in the right ventricle, may advance into the pulmonary artery, or may retract into the right atrium. Rarely the tip will perforate the wall of the ventricle and lodge outside the heart. This may cause the pacemaker to capture the diaphragm (which gives the patient hiccups at the rate set on the pulse generator, ventricular tachycardia, or ventricular fibrillation).

Another cause of loss of capture: ischemia of the myocardium or fibrosis near the tip. Ischemic tissue has a higher threshold and, so, needs more energy to depolarize the myocardium and produce a contraction. Some rarer causes: The negative terminal of the pulse generator becomes disconnected from the distal wire of the pacing catheter; or the power cable or catheter breaks.

What to do about loss of capture? Turn the patient on his left side, which may let the catheter fall back in contact with the right ventricle wall. Turn up the setting of the output dial. If ischemic myocardium is the cause, the increased amperage may compensate for it.

Sensing: If the patient's apical pulse is higher than the rate set on the pulse generator, but the sense-pace dial shows

change the patient's position, the battery, or the pacemaker unit. Notify the doctor.

• When discontinuing the pacemaker, turn the rate down *gradually* to avoid causing asystole.

PERMANENT PACEMAKER
• Teach the patient and family how to count and record his pulse daily.

• Explain the signs of battery failure: change in pacing rate, dizziness, Stokes-Adams attacks, dyspnea, or increased weight gain.

• Have the patient watch for signs of infection or skin breakdown.

• Tell him when to notify the doctor: when pulse rate changes; symptoms recur; he has signs of infection; or has suffered a blow that may have damaged his pacemaker.

• Make sure the patient understands the necessity of follow-up care at regular intervals.

continuous firing at the lower rate, the pacer is not sensing the patient's own heart rate. The pacer should never fire when the patient's own rate consistently exceeds the pacer's set rate. In this situation, called competition, the pacer is competing with the patient's own pacemaker for control of his heart instead of assisting it. This causes an irregular heart rhythm. Competition is dangerous because it may cause ventricular fibrillation if the pacer fires during the myocardium's recovery or repolarization phase, at the top of the T wave.

What causes it? Most likely, the catheter tip has moved so that the sensing electrode doesn't receive a strong enough signal from the patient's myocardium. Indeed, the tip may be displaced so much that both sensing and capture are lost. Again, other causes include broken or disconnected wiring. What to do? Turn the patient on his left side, which may move the pacing catheter back into place. Check the demand dial to make sure it is in the full demand position. If neither of these procedures restores proper function, and if the patient's own rate is adequate to maintain circulation, turn the pacemaker off to prevent ventricular fibrillation and call the doctor at once to reposition the catheter. Be prepared to begin CPR in case of complete heart block.

Patient-teaching vital

When a temporary pacemaker is stopped, be sure that the patient does not feel any anxiety about its being discontinued. If he does, reassure him. When a patient with a temporary pacemaker is to get a permanent one, explain how he will live with his new equipment. Usually, the interval between temporary and permanent implantations is long enough to allow a relaxed period of preparation.

Some patients try to deny that they must depend on a mechanical device to resume a useful, active life. If such denial becomes a problem, the patient may benefit from a visit from another patient who already has a permanent pacemaker. If he still resists, he may need psychiatric consultation. His persistent denial will only mean that sooner or later he will harm himself by not following instructions. When he cooperates, discuss his return to active life (see insert, *Questions Patients Ask*). Be sure he understands: Life with a pacemaker may not be the life he led 10 years earlier, but it can and should be better than the life he could have without it.

SKILLCHECK 2

1. How does hypertension predispose to coronary artery disease?

2. Why do patients with angina frequently experience pain in the left shoulder and arm?

3. Which of the following patients is most at risk for a pulmonary embolus: a 42-year-old male in CCU, 3 days postmyocardial infarction; a 16-year-old male 6 days after knee surgery; a 31-year-old obese primipara, 5 days postCaesarean section; a 28-year-old male immobilized in traction for 36 days following a motorcycle accident.

4. Martha is a 56-year-old woman who has been hospitalized for a fractured pelvis for the past 24 days. You notice that her respirations have suddenly gone from 16/min. to 32/min., although her color is unchanged. She is complaining of chest pain and looks very apprehensive. Her blood pressure is unchanged, but her pulse is 116/min. regular and her temperature is 100.4° F. (38° C.). She had rales in both bases but no S_3 or S_4. What's the most likely explanation for her symptoms? What should you do?

5. John is a 38-year-old black male who comes to your clinic because of fatigue and early morning headaches. On ophthalmoscopy you notice soft exudates, hemorrhages, and papilledema. What condition do these findings suggest and what is John's probable prognosis?

6. The most specific serum enzyme study used to diagnose an AMI is: CPK, CPK-MB, SGOT, or LDH?

7. Which of these EKG findings is *not* typical of an AMI: Deep Q waves, S-T elevation, S-T depression, or T wave inversion?

8. How does Inderal reduce myocardial oxygen consumption?

9. Tom Beal has just been admitted to your unit to "Rule out AMI." He had chest pain at home 4 hours ago, received morphine sulfate, 4 mg I.V., in the E.D., and is now complaining of nausea and is vomiting. What is happening? What should you watch for?

10. On auscultation you notice that Tom's heart sounds are abnormal: There are 3 sounds instead of 2. What does this mean? Should you call his doctor?

11. Tom is asking for something for pain. Should you give the medication (Demerol 75 mg.) I.M. or I.V.?

12. John Anderson is a patient on your unit who is 6 days post MI. He's been recovering uneventfully. When you bring in his evening medication you find him unresponsive. His vital signs are: BP 90/60, P 154/min., R 32/min. You notice that his BP varies 15 mm Hg with respiration (pulsus paradoxus). He is lying at a 45° angle but his neck veins are distended to 20 cm. What has happened?

(Answers on page 171)

IN THE ELDERLY:

EXPECT VASCULAR DETERIORATION

15

Peripheral Vascular Disease
Cause of leg pain

BY IDABELLE REAM, RN

UNLESS YOUR NURSING CARE involves only the very young, you probably often hear patients complain of aching legs. Elderly patients are especially likely to complain of cramps, fullness, and aching in the legs. Do you dismiss such complaints lightly? Or do you consider them a likely sign of peripheral vascular disease ... of arterial or venous insufficiency? Both can lead to progressive suffering and disability unless they're promptly and correctly managed.

Peripheral vascular disease can be arterial, venous, or both, so you need to know the differences between them. Let's look at *arterial* disease first.

Chronic arterial insufficiency (arteriosclerosis obliterans [ASO] is most common) causes pain in one or both legs. It forces the patient to stop walking until the pain goes away. He'll usually describe the pain as sharp — like a stabbing knife or a vise squeezing the leg. Or he may describe a feeling of unusual tiredness in one leg as he walks. Such a feeling is apt to be brought on by some change in activity pattern; for example, a new job that requires more walking than before. This new exertion calls attention to a condition that may have existed for years.

ASO: What patients need to know

Arteriosclerosis obliterans (ASO) causes the walls of large and medium-sized peripheral arteries to thicken, harden, and lose their elasticity. As the lumen narrows, the blood flow decreases and blood clots may form. When collateral circulation cannot compensate for the block, ischemia results. The ASO patient, age 50 or older, will feel a knife-like pain during exercise, proximal to the blockage. In advanced cases, pain may occur even during rest.

Have your ASO patients follow this checklist of do's and don'ts:
DO:
• Wash feet daily and wear clean, well-fitting socks.
• Trim nails straight across, but not too closely.
• Clean small cuts carefully with mild soap and water, and protect from further injury.
• Call the doctor to report any persistent leg problem.
DON'T:
• Don't go barefoot.
• Don't let your legs become extremely cold.
• Don't wear clothes that constrict your legs or feet.
• Don't let your legs get sunburned.
• Don't cut or file corns or calluses. Don't use chemical corn and callus remedies.
• Don't put a hot water bottle, heat lamp, or heating pad directly on the affected area. Instead, put the heat on the lower back or abdomen. This will warm the legs in about 15 minutes.

So your assessment should include specific questions such as, "Do your legs hurt you while you're walking?" or "Do you ever have any sharp pain in your legs?" Also, ask how long such pain usually lasts. In patients with arterial insufficiency, leg pain induced by walking subsides quickly if the patient stands still for a few minutes. But if the pain persists for more than a few minutes after resting, or if it forces the patient to sit down or elevate his leg to relieve the pain, he may have some other disease. Possibilities: neuropathy or osteoarthritis. Incidentally, remember to ask elderly patients about leg pain even if they don't complain of it; many consider such pain normal at their age and not worth mentioning.

As ASO progresses and ischemia becomes severe, the patient experiences pain even *without exercising*. He is apt to feel the pain first in the toes, heel, and dorsum of his foot. He'll probably describe such pain as a severe throbbing or ache that wakes him up after he's been in bed several hours. The pain may be increased by cold or elevation of the affected foot. For relief, he may have to rub his foot, hang it over the edge of the bed, or walk around the room.

A sensation of burning or cold often accompanies the pain of advanced ASO. This may also be a sign of diabetic or alcoholic neuropathy. But with ASO you'll be able to feel the cold yourself — and probably notice a diminished or absent pulse as well. With neuropathy, the foot feels warm and distal pulses are usually good.

How bad is it?

The patient's description of his leg problems can tell you the severity of arterial occlusion. If he says he can walk only about three or four city blocks without rest, he must have significant occlusion with little collateral circulation. A patient with only mild disease can walk three times as far.

To further gauge the degree of insufficiency, ask the patient to lie on his back. Taking his heels in the palm of your hand, raise both legs about 2 feet above the bed for about a minute. Then, look for color changes in the skin of both feet and legs, particularly on the soles. (With dark-skinned patients, look at the soles and plantar surface of the toes.) If circulation is good, the normal pink color will diminish only slightly. If not, pallor will develop, according to the degree of occlusion. If ischemia is severe, the entire leg may become pale.

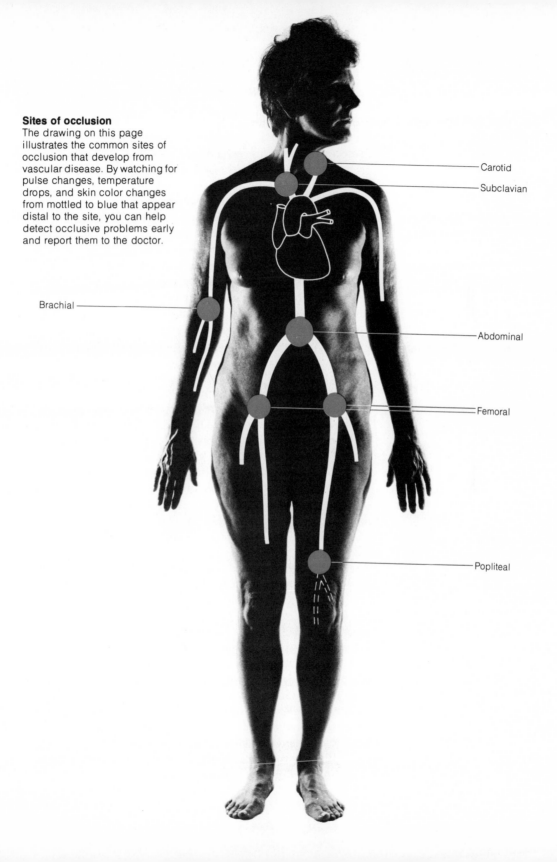

Sites of occlusion
The drawing on this page illustrates the common sites of occlusion that develop from vascular disease. By watching for pulse changes, temperature drops, and skin color changes from mottled to blue that appear distal to the site, you can help detect occlusive problems early and report them to the doctor.

Carotid

Subclavian

Brachial

Abdominal

Femoral

Popliteal

Varicose veins: What patients need to know

Varicose veins — dilated superficial leg veins — are believed to result from man's upright stance: The condition has never been found in quadrupeds.

Varicosities result from defects in the venous valves, which normally prevent retrograde blood flow. First, the proximal valves in the legs fail, increasing the column of blood that must be supported by the distal veins. The increased hydrostatic pressure distends the veins, giving them their characteristic knotlike appearance. The increased pressure may cause the capillaries to rupture, producing petechiae.

Exercise "pumps" the blood through the veins and prevents pooling. Thus the venous pressure is much lower in an active person.

To help alleviate the swelling and discomfort of varicose veins, advise your patients to:

• Avoid prolonged sitting or standing. If you must remain seated, elevate your legs whenever possible. On long car trips, stop hourly for a brief walk. If you must stand for a long time, exercise legs by periodically rising on tiptoes and shifting weight from foot to foot.

• Take a long walk daily — up to 2 miles if possible — wearing elastic bandages or stockings. Use stairs instead of elevators. Swim whenever possible.

• Never wear anything that constricts circulation such as garters or knee stockings.

• Elevate legs above heart level for an hour a day.

• Protect your legs from injury.

• Maintain a diet to prevent obesity.

If you notice pallor in *both* legs, chances are the patient has an aorto-iliac block or bilateral arterial blocks in both legs. You can confirm this by having him sit up quickly and dangle his legs over the edge of the bed. The time required for color to return to the feet indicates arterial patency. With normal circulation, color returns to the feet in 10 seconds or less and superficial veins fill in 10 to 15 seconds. With significant blockage, color returns after 40 to 60 seconds; with severe blockage, after 1 to 2 minutes.

Some ASO patients may need angiography to evaluate the need for surgery. Usual indications are:

• severe intermittent claudication that handicaps the patient physically, economically, or socially

• a sudden decrease in claudication distance

• skin changes caused by severe arterial insufficiency (including ulcers).

Preventing progression

Arterial insufficiency is not reversible, but the patient — with your guidance — can do much to prevent progression of the disease to avoid complications that might require surgery, to reduce pain, and to increase his endurance.

According to some authorities, more than a third of the amputations due to complications of ASO result directly or indirectly from chemical, mechanical, or thermal injury. This means the patient must learn to take continuing meticulous care of his legs and know how to improve circulation. He must learn to...

• *stop smoking*. This is most important! Tobacco contains powerful vasoconstrictors that further decrease circulation and often increase pain.

• *sleep with the head of his bed raised* 4 to 6 inches on wooden blocks.

• *avoid injury*. The ischemic limb is at high risk for bacterial infections, which may start with the tiniest break in the skin. "Babying" the affected leg must become second nature. (See page 156 for some do's and don'ts that will help.)

• *develop collateral circulation*. Walking is the best way to increase collateral circulation and claudication distance. Instruct the patient to walk at least 30 minutes two or three times daily. He can rest during the walk, but not the instant he begins to feel discomfort. He should walk until pain forces him to stop. When the pain goes away, he should resume walking.

Some patients become discouraged because, at first, their claudication distance decreases rather than increases. Assure them that this is common. The distance they can walk will depend on various things: temperature, walking surface, grade, and others. Nevertheless, if they persist, they will soon be walking twice as far as before without needing to rest.

Recognizing venous disorders

Some patients who complain of leg pain and fatigue may have venous insufficiency rather than arterial. The usual clues to venous involvement are:

- swollen superficial veins
- a full or tight feeling in the affected leg or legs
- leg cramps at night
- early fatigue of the leg
- leg pain during the menstrual period
- nodules or ropelike formations palpable in the legs
- swollen calves or thighs.

Certain management techniques for varicose veins are contraindicated for arterial insufficiency. So be sure these two disorders don't coexist before suggesting treatments. They often do, especially in elderly and diabetic patients. Here again, taking a good history will help. What's the most telling difference? Walking relieves venous symptoms; but it brings on claudication in patients with arterial insufficiency.

Surgery is now largely outmoded for treatment of varicosities, particularly primary (superficial) ones. Phlebography provides the best way to distinguish between primary varicosities (involving superficial veins only) and secondary varicosities (involving deep veins — deep thrombophlebitis). But other clues may help too. If the patient's history shows that the condition has developed slowly (over several years) and he has led a fairly active life, chances are that deep veins are involved. If the patient has led a sedentary life recently, or has work that requires prolonged standing on his feet (such as a waitress or sales clerk), chances favor superficial vein involvement. A family history of varicose veins also suggests superficial varicosity.

Managing mild varicosities

Uncomplicated cases of varicose veins can be managed well

SUPERFICIAL VS. DEEP THROMBOPHLEBITIS

Forming a thrombus

A century ago, a German pathologist named Rudolf Virchow identified the conditions that predispose to thrombus formation: hypercoagulability of the blood; alterations in the integrity of blood vessel walls; and venous stasis.

Hypercoagulability of the blood is associated with:
- pregnancy and oral contraceptive use
- postoperative states
- fever
- sickle cell anemia
- certain malignancies (especially of the pancreas)
- polycythemia vera
- abnormal "stickiness" of the platelets
- myocardial infarction
- abrupt discontinuation of anticoagulants (rebound hypercoagulability).

Unfortunately, little can be done to prevent hypercoagulability other than to teach patients who take anticoagulants not to discontinue them without a doctor's supervision.

Changes in the vessel wall may result from:
- trauma
- peripheral vascular disease
- degenerative diseases
- vein distention (as of the uterine vein during pregnancy)
- pooling of the blood (as happens when the body holds one position too long).

Venous stasis results from clots caused by:
- obesity
- congestive heart failure
- arrhythmias (atrial fibrillation can cause thrombus formation in the right atrium)
- long-term immobility.

Researchers have identified the population most likely to develop a thrombus:
- women, particularly the obese
- people with a history of venous thrombosis
- people whose occupations require prolonged sitting or standing
- patients on bedrest
- postop patients
- the elderly.

Know the differences between superficial and deep thrombophlebitis, so you can make a rapid, accurate assessment. Since these two conditions require different treatments, learn how to recognize the clinical distinctions and how to help the patient implement his care.

Superficial

SYMPTOMS: *Aching and swelling* usually localized into a "knot" or "bump." You can usually palpate a firm mass along the course of a superficial vein. Although this condition accompanies more symptoms than deep thrombosis, it's actually less dangerous because there's less chance of embolization.

Differential diagnosis

Insect bites (Check for history of exposure, itching, and locations away from known course of superficial vein.)
Cellulitis and abscesses (marked tenderness and fluctuance)
Subcutaneous hematoma (history of trauma, location)

USUAL LOCATION
Leg or arm. Often above or below a palpable varicose vein.

TREATMENT
Symptomatic relief for duration of symptoms, usually 2 to 3 days. Hot baths or compresses, elastic support. Avoidance of stasis: Walk or elevate legs.
Anti-inflammatory drugs, such as phenylbutazone (Butazolidin).

Deep

SYMPTOMS: *Pain* varying in degree from severe cramping to a feeling of heaviness. The patient's leg will usually feel tender. *Swelling,* the most reliable sign, may be detected only with careful bilateral measurements. (Some experts recommend that all surgery patients be measured pre- and postoperatively at thigh, calf, and ankle to detect phlebothrombosis. This "silent" thrombosis often goes unrecognized before embolization, simply because no inflammation of the vein wall is involved.)
Homan's sign — calf pain during dorsiflexion of the foot, may be present but is not reliable.
Ramirez test — Have patient flex his knee. Calf pain is positive sign when you inflate a BP cuff above knee to 40 mm Hg.

Differential diagnosis

Muscle tear (Check for history of trauma, sharp pain on exertion, ecchymosis over calf and below malleoli.)
Knee joint effusion (ballottement of patella)
Cellulitis (leukocytosis, high fever, erythema)

USUAL LOCATION
Calf vein is most common. Forty percent of patients develop thrombi bilaterally.
Femoral vein, frequently in combination with calf vein.
Iliofemoral thrombus: iliac and femoral veins.
Less common: pelvic vein and upper extremities.

TREATMENT
Prevention of emboli; bedrest and elevation of involved extremity; anticoagulation; surgical thrombectomy if thrombus occludes a major vein.

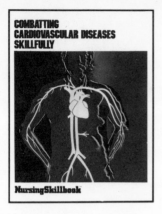

**COMBATTING
CARDIOVASCULAR DISEASES
SKILLFULLY**

NursingSkillbook

The authoritative book on cardiovascular disease "Combating Cardiovascular Diseases Skillfully," only $8.95 each.

Cardiovascular nursing no longer means just the care of patients in the coronary care unit. Besides direct nursing care, nurses are expected to promote health and prevent cardiovascular disease in many ways.

To participate in health care, you must have highly developed skills in physical assessment, history taking, diagnostic test interpretation and health teaching.

Among the many aspects of cardiovascular nursing included are:
Cardiovascular assessment/Cardiac babies/Cardiac surgery/
Hypertension/Coronary artery disease/Congestive failure/
Cardiac complications/Peripheral vascular disease/Aneurysm

There are sections on advice to patients — rehabilitation — emergency cardiovascular drugs. No matter where you work or how developed your skills, this book will help improve your care in nursing the patient with cardiovascular disease.

Please send _____ copies of "Combating Cardiovascular Diseases Skillfully," at $8.95

Name _____

Address _____

City _____

State or
Province _____

Zip or
Mail code _____

Pa. residents please add 6% sales tax.
Offer valid in U.S. and Canada only. Elsewhere, orders must include prepayment of $8.95 (U.S. funds) for each copy ordered. Allow 8 weeks for overseas delivery.

AI09

FREE shipping and handling on prepaid orders.

Nursing Skillbook series

Examine these books for 10 days free... Nursing Skillbook series
You'll save $1.00 on every book you buy.

The Skillbook you're holding is part of an exciting series...you can examine each title for 10 days *free* and save $1.00 on each book you buy. Membership in the Nursing Skillbook series is guaranteed to help you improve your nursing skills. With these valuable books, you'll: □ Test your reactions to difficult situations in nursing...such as working with a patient who does not know his illness is terminal...and compare these reactions with opinions of authorities. □ Discover new ways of dealing with trying tasks, such as deciding whether an EKG is really normal or not. □ Marvel at the human body's ways of informing you that something's wrong, as in nonketotic acidosis. □ Find fresh insights into complicated subjects, like hypernatremia and hyperkalemia. □ Prize some of the comprehensive lists included, such as the nature and side effects of all the cancer drugs available today. □ Much more.

Each handsome volume offers: ● 192 fact- and illustration-filled pages ● Convenient 7½" by 9" size ● Durable hardcover binding ● 68,000 words of authoritative, useful text ● SKILLCHECKS, a learning method that helps you use the books' wealth of information in daily practice.

□ **Yes, I would like to examine the first volume of the Nursing Skillbook series.** If I decide to keep it, I will pay $7.95 plus shipping and handling. I then will receive future volumes shipped one at a time every 2 to 3 months. Each costs $7.95 plus shipping and handling (10-day, free-examination basis). There is no minimum number of books that I must buy, and I may cancel my subscription at any time.

Name _____

Address _____

City _____

State or
Province _____

Zip or
Mail code _____

Offer valid in U.S. and Canada only.

SER09

PLEASE DETACH THIS STUB BEFORE MAILING

FIRST CLASS
PERMIT NO. 1903
HICKSVILLE, N.Y

BUSINESS REPLY MAIL

No Postage Stamp Necessary if Mailed in the United States

Postage will be paid by:

6 Commercial Street
Hicksville, N.Y. 11801

FIRST CLASS
PERMIT NO. 1903
HICKSVILLE, N.Y

BUSINESS REPLY MAIL

No Postage Stamp Necessary if Mailed in the United States

Postage will be paid by:

6 Commercial Street
Hicksville, N.Y. 11801

with elastic stockings and bandages. By pressing in on the legs, the elastic counteracts swelling and supports the vein walls, aiding blood-flow to the heart. Some patients prefer Ace bandages, because they can concentrate the most support to a small area where it's needed most. Whether they use stockings or bandages, patients should put them on before getting out of bed (before the leg has a chance to swell). And they should take them off before retiring, unless the doctor prescribes their nighttime use.

Not surprisingly, many patients, particularly young women, hate to wear support hose. Luckily, many of them can get adequate support from medium-weight elastic pantyhose and still be fashionable. In fact, patients with mild varicose veins can even wear standard hosiery for a few hours during social occasions without ill effects.

Patients disturbed by "spider veins" (telangiectases) can hide them easily with special cosmetics made to hide severe blemishes. Certainly, cosmetics are safer than treatment with injections of sclerosing agents. Such injections are generally only temporarily effective anyway and may lead to complications.

Dealing with stasis complications
Stasis dermatitis, induration, and ulcers sometimes result from chronic venous insufficiency. Dermatitis and induration usually heal with simple treatments: local applications of warm, moist dressings and nonirritating ointments and creams; bed rest; and elevation of the legs. Stasis ulcers are usually more serious. Before treating stasis ulcers, you must be sure that they are indeed stasis and not ischemic. This distinction is vital for patients with both arterial and venous insufficiency. Such patients need special consideration. With them, you must maintain a delicate balance — constraining the venous circulation without disrupting the arterial. That's difficult but possible.

Edema indicates the need for elastic support, but not too much. The stocking should be a lightweight type. Or, in many cases, a 4 to 6 inch elastic bandage will work better because it can be wrapped more loosely. Whatever support is selected, the patient should remove it at the first sign of any pain, then reapply it after a rest period. Sometimes, cutting the top and toe from an elastic stocking will provide the support needed

Two ischemic conditions
Two vascular diseases, Raynaud's disease and Buerger's disease, may cause ischemia, from cyanosis to gangrene.

Raynaud's disease, an idiopathic hypersensitivity to cold, affects the hands more than the feet and women more than men. Attacks may be reversible, or irreversible, involving necrosis, atrophy of the nails, and osteoporosis of the fingers and toes.

Raynaud's disease can be treated symptomatically or, in severe cases, with sympathectomy.

Buerger's disease (thromboangiitis obliterans, pictured above), nonatheromatous lesions of small arteries, veins, and nerves, affects the lower extremities predominantly. The involved part suffers cold, postural color changes, pain, superficial migratory phlebitis, arteriolar spasms, and even gangrene. Doctors treat the disease symptomatically.

Patients with Buerger's or Raynaud's disease who stop smoking relieve the vaso-constriction that smoking produces.

Treating stasis ulcers

Venous insufficiency can cause painless stasis ulcers on the medial aspect of the leg. Most will require bedrest. Small ulcers can be treated by compression with an Unna boot bandage.

A stasis ulcer should be painted with gentian violet 1% and mild topical antibiotics, if infected, and then covered with sterile dressing. The bandage must be changed every 7 to 10 days and kept dry. To keep clean the patient should take sponge baths. If pain or seepage develops, the dressing should be changed immediately.

Stasis ulcers heal in 6 to 12 weeks. After the compression treatment, the patient should wear elastic stockings to prevent recurrence.

without restricting arterial flow. A patient who has edema and stasis symptoms, or one who's recovering from thrombophlebitis, probably needs a tailor-made heavyweight support stocking. You should examine the fit of such elastic stockings to ensure the right degree of support.

A patient with both venous and arterial insufficiency should sleep on a level bed. That is because elevating the feet will reduce edema, but will also reduce arterial flow; elevating the head will increase arterial flow, but increase edema. Even better than a level bed is an *oscillating* bed, if available. Its gradual rocking reduces edema without impairing arterial circulation.

Counsel life-long care

Once they develop, peripheral vascular diseases are usually chronic. Thus, the most important service you can offer these patients is this: Convince them of the need to continue special management after their immediate problem has been cleared up. For example, they should maintain a regular exercise program. Many elderly patients are all too willing to accept discomfort and disability as the inevitable price of growing old. However, if they remain conscientious about their leg care, they can look forward to steadily increased endurance and mobility. They can thereby maintain freedom and self-sufficiency.

16

Aneurysm
Potentially fatal defect

BY GAIL D'ONOFRIO LONG, RN, MS

IF YOU MUST CARE for an aneurysm patient, you may have trouble on your hands. First of all, given the typical age group of such patients (60 to 70), you must be on the lookout for signs of pulmonary impairment and even cerebral complications of atherosclerosis. Then, because the surgical repair of the condition requires a massive incision — from xiphoid to pubis — the patient can easily bleed and leak fluid. Here's what to expect in (and do for) such a patient.

Chances are — by four to one — that your patient with an abdominal aortic aneurysm (AAA) will be a man like Sidney Rosoff, a 63-year-old math teacher with atherosclerosis. Mr. Rosoff's annual physical exam revealed a pulsatile mass in the midabdominal region. When questioned, the only symptom he admitted was a dull epigastric pain and a feeling of fullness after meals. But he'd assumed it was indigestion.

Mr. Rosoff's case is not unusual. In fact, more than half the people with an aneurysm have no symptoms. When symptoms do occur, they arise from the aneurysm's pressure on surrounding structures, from its stretching of the mesenteric root, or from slow leakage of blood causing retroperitoneal pressure.

A baleful bulge
This arteriogram shows an
abdominal aortic aneurysm
before surgery. The aneurysm
does not extend to the renal
arteries, but the widening of the
aorta to its bifurcation does
suggest the involvement of the
iliac arteries.

What causes an arterial
aneurysm? In 95% of cases, the
characteristic bulge in the arterial
wall results from atherosclerosis.
But it can stem instead from
trauma, congenital defect,
syphilis, cystic medionecrosis, or
nonspecific inflammation.

What's common to all
aneurysms is damage to the
middle or muscular layer of the
vessel, the tunica media. With the
media's incompetence, the inner
(intima) and outer (adventitia)
layers of the artery are also
helplessly stretched outward.
Pressure of the coursing blood as
it pounds against the defect can
not only enlarge the aneurysm, by
exerting relentless pressure on
the weakened vessel walls. It can
also wear away surrounding
structures. In fact, wear and tear
on the vessel will ultimately cause
its rupture.

Patients with symptoms most commonly complain of pain in
the lumbar region radiating into the flank or groin. Such pain
stems from pressure on the lumbar nerves. Depending on the
atherosclerotic involvement of distal arteries — the iliac and
femoral — the patient may complain of symptoms produced
by arterial ischemia or occlusion, such as claudication. He
may also have abdominal pulsations, GI discomfort, changes
in bowel habits, or peripheral edema.

Luckily, 80% of all abdominal aneurysms *are* palpable, so
any time you examine an older patient, especially one with
vascular disease, keep this in mind. A flat plate of Mr.
Rosoff's abdomen revealed a 5-centimeter aneurysm (a
threatening size) with a calcified wall. Since an untreated
aneurysm inevitably grows larger, the doctor recommended
surgical resection to avoid a potentially fatal rupture.

Rupture?

How do you recognize rupture of an abdominal aneurysm into
the peritoneum? Its chief clinical features are pain and signs of
blood loss. Many victims feel a sudden and then constant
severe pain in the abdomen, or pain in the lower back, radiating to the groin. Along with the pain come weakness, sweating, tachycardia, and a drop in blood pressure, either mild or
severe enough to signal shock.

If you palpate such a patient's abdomen, you'll no longer
feel a discrete aneurysmal wall. Instead, you'll feel a pulsatile
heave of the entire retroperitoneum. There won't be time for
tests. Once the diagnosis is made, the patient must be rushed
to the operating room. No attempt can be made to stabilize
him, nor can surgery be further postponed. If treated in time,
the patient's chances of surviving are about 3 to 2. If not, he
will die.

Who's a candidate for surgery? Patients with a lesion less
than 6 cm may be treated conservatively (with regular echog-
raphy to detect enlargement). Even so, the potential for rupture in a "small" aneurysm can still be as high as 20%. With an
aneurysm larger than 6 cm, the risk of rupture is from 40% to
80% within 2 to 5 years of diagnosis. Since aneurysms tend to
enlarge, most vascular surgeons recommend resection in all
relatively good-risk patients with an aneurysm larger than 6
cm, and in those under 65 with an aneurysm between 4 and 6
cm. A symptomatic aneurysm, of course, warrants immediate

Areas of alarm
Aneurysms tend to occur at or near an arterial bifurcation and most commonly affect the abdominal aorta. You can see the common sites in this illustration.

Internal carotid artery

Arch of the aorta

Ascending aorta

Descending thoracic aorta

Superior mesenteric artery

Thoracicoabdominal segment of the aorta

Abdominal aorta

Femoral artery

Popliteal artery

consideration for surgery.

In cases where a rupture is not imminent, however, elective surgery allows time for completion of diagnostic preop tests.

Preop management

The day before elective surgery is filled with tests, consultations, and numerous procedures. Your preop role with aneurysm patients can be strong: obtaining baseline data (vital signs, the character of peripheral pulses, breath sounds, and so on), taking a history, explaining the various procedures involved, and offering the patient and his family support to reduce their anxiety.

Before Mr. Rosoff was taken to the O.R. we took a complete set of vital signs and inserted an I.V. and a Foley catheter. We weighed him on the ICU bed scale to obtain a baseline weight: Any change would guide fluid management (a crucial consideration before, during, and after surgery). An arterial line and a central venous pressure (CVP) line were inserted. If the patient has heart disease, a pulmonary artery catheter allows continuous monitoring of PAP and PWP. Remember that CVP monitoring measures right heart pressure and may not accurately reflect pressure on the left side of the heart. Along with other preop medications, we gave him cephalothin (Keflin), a broad-spectrum antibiotic, which would be continued for 48 hours postoperatively to prevent infection.

Postop management complex

In the O.R., the surgeon resected the aneurysm and inserted a Dacron bifurcation graft. It extended from below the renal arteries to the femoral arteries. Mr. Rosoff was transferred to the ICU with an endotracheal tube, a Salem sump nasogastric tube, a CVP line, an arterial line, and a Foley catheter all in place. We hung an I.V., with 5% dextrose in ½ normal saline with 20 mEq potassium. Then we placed him on a MA-1 volume-controlled ventilator, and connected him to the cardiac monitor. We sent blood for a complete blood count, electrolytes, BUN, creatinine, and ABGs. Then we started an ICU flow sheet to monitor and record his vital signs and his hemodynamic, respiratory, and neurologic status, as well as his fluid intake and output.

Our next job: to take a complete set of Mr. Rosoff's vital signs. His rectal temperature on admission to the ICU was

Aneurysms take many forms
Damage to the media layer may cause the aneurysm to bulge on only one side of the artery. This kind is called saccular.

If an aneurysm bulges out on both sides of the affected vessel, it's called a fusiform aneurysm.

99.4° F. (37.4° C.); heart rate, 94; blood pressure, 120/60; and CVP, 10 cm H_2O. (To prevent the "declamping hypotension phenomenon" the patient's vascular volume is kept to the maximum point on his Starling curve during surgery.) We checked his popliteal, pedal, and posterior tibial pulses every hour at first, recording them on the flow sheet. We also noted the temperature, color, and movement of his legs. (A decreased or absent pulse along with cool, mottled extremities would have indicated embolization — or even occlusion of the graft.) Also, to watch for internal bleeding, we measured and recorded his abdominal girth every 2 hours.

Fortunately, renal failure — once a common complication of abdominal aneurysm resection — is now rare. But you need to know the urine output just to ensure adequate renal perfusion. If it's less than 30 ml per hour for 2 consecutive hours, notify the doctor. Check the urine for specific gravity at least every 3 or 4 hours. If the patient becomes hypovolemic, his kidneys will try to conserve salt and water by producing only small amounts of concentrated urine. Its specific gravity will be more than 1.030. Mr. Rosoff's urine reached a specific gravity of 1.025, high normal.

Blood splitting vessel layers, a dissecting aneurysm, commonly affects the thoracic aorta. It's associated with connective tissue disorders or trauma.

We checked for evidence of emboli in his legs due to necrotic debris and monitored the EKG carefully, watching for changes consistent with ischemia. In older patients with atherosclerosis, like Mr. Rosoff, the potential for CVA means that you must check neurologic vital signs not only in the initial assessment but also every 2 to 3 hours thereafter. About an hour after admission to the ICU, Mr. Rosoff was awake, alert, and oriented. He showed an equal reaction to light in his pupils, had a good grip in either hand, and remained stable.

Respiratory care crucial

Because many such patients have a history of pulmonary disease, possibly because of their age, you must assess their respiratory status frequently. You must be proficient in auscultating breath sounds and identifying any adventitious sounds such as rales, which may denote fluid in the alveoli.

Many aneurysm patients develop respiratory distress from wet lung syndrome 24 to 48 hours postoperatively. This seems to result from an inflammatory response to the massive resection, which builds a large amount of fluid in the retroperitoneal space. A day or two postop, this fluid may start leaking into the

When all vessel layers rupture, as in trauma, this is called a false aneurysm. (A true aneurysm has one layer intact.) Escaping blood forms a pulsating hematoma.

Resecting an aneurysm
Repair of an abdominal aortic aneurysm starts with a midline incision made from the xiphoid process to the pubis. The bowel is then displaced, and another incision in the peritoneum exposes the aneurysm. Most times, the aneurysm begins below the level of the renal arteries, which aren't involved. For that reason, blood flow to the kidneys generally need not be impaired when the surgeon clamps the aorta. Although the inferior mesenteric artery *is* commonly involved in the aneurysm, in most cases it's simply tied off.

When the surgeon begins working on the defect itself, he splits the aneurysm and cleans it of all clots and atherosclerotic material. Then, he anastomoses a preclotted bifurcated sleeve of Dacron to the *inner* walls of the aorta above and below the defect.

The surgeon then closes the aneurysm wall over the graft. This serves as an extra protective layer between the graft and viscera. And it prevents complications such as an aortoduodenal fistula.

interstitial spaces of the lung. But usually this complication can be prevented with a diuretic such as furosemide (Lasix).

We were careful to turn Mr. Rosoff every 2 hours, suction his endotracheal tube as needed, and take blood for gas determinations at regular intervals. Besides an EKG, we took a chest X-ray as soon as possible after surgery, and repeated it daily while he was in the ICU. Mr. Rosoff assisted the respirator minimally. We suctioned him for moderate amounts of white sputum. Breath sounds were present bilaterally, and we heard a few bibasilar rales. We were eager to avoid respiratory alkalosis from overuse of the ventilator. Such alkalosis would increase the affinity of oxygen for the hemoglobin molecule and so impede its use by the tissues. Mr. Rosoff's blood gases were normal: PO_2, 126; PCO_2, 38; pH, 7.45. We adjusted the FIO_2 on the ventilator accordingly.

Most aneurysm repair patients remain intubated for 24 hours after surgery. They can be extubated and started on oxygen by mask when they can generate an adequate tidal volume, vital capacity, peak inspiratory force...and when their ABGs are normal while being weaned from the ventilator. Then they need chest physiotherapy, nasotracheal suction, and early mobilization. Help them by giving pain medication beforehand and by splinting the huge incision with pillows during coughing exercises.

After aneurysm repair, patients need a nasogastric tube to keep the stomach and duodenum decompressed. This eases any pressure on the suture line and reveals bleeding in the upper GI tract. If your patient has a tube, check routinely to be sure it's patent. Record the amount of drainage and the results of the guaiac test. The nasogastric tube remains in place for 3 to 5 days after surgery because paralytic ileus can easily occur anytime in this period. Once you hear bowel sounds and the patient passes gas by rectum, the tube can be withdrawn and the patient started on a liquid diet. The activity schedule for patients with aneurysm repair varies. We had Mr. Rosoff out of bed by the second postop day. During the first week, we had him avoid sitting to prevent pressure on the graft, and avoid dangling his legs to prevent edema. We taught him breathing exercises, his activity schedule, and the low-fat, low-cholesterol diet his doctor had prescribed. Once discharged from the ICU, his activities were continually increased. He went home in good condition 10 days after surgery.

SKILLCHECK 3

1. A 67-year-old retired lawyer, Mike Loger, is a patient on your unit. He tells you that he has pain in both legs after walking 6 to 8 blocks. His pain goes away within a few minutes after he rests. Would you suspect: arterial insufficiency, venous insufficiency, osteoarthritis, or neuropathy?

2. How can you confirm Mr. Loger's diagnosis and assess his degree of insufficiency?

3. Marie Wade has been a waitress for the past 23 years. She has just been admitted to your unit for an evaluation of her varicose veins. Do you think her varicosities are superficial or deep? How can you make the distinction?

4. Which of the following symptoms indicates venous insufficiency: leg cramps at night; leg pain (claudication) after walking 6 to 8 blocks that is relieved by resting for a brief period of time; nodules or ropelike formation in the legs; or painful swelling in the calves?

5. What relieves venous symptoms? Smoking, resting, walking, or dangling the legs?

6. What causes leg ulcers? Ischemia secondary to arterial insufficiency; stasis secondary to venous insufficiency; or both?

7. How are abdominal aneurysms detectable? By auscultation, by palpation, by inspection, or by percussion?

8. Abdominal aneurysms are most likely to occur in persons...over 60; 40 to 60; under 40?

9. What causes arterial aneurysms?

10. True or false: When all vessel layers rupture, this is called a fusiform aneurysm.

(Answers on page 172)

SKILLCHECK ANSWERS

ANSWERS TO SKILLCHECK 1 (page 41)

Situation 1
Sally has a waterhammer or Corrigan's pulse. It probably indicates patent ductus arteriosus (PDA), although it's also found with aortic regurgitation.

Situation 2
In children the diastolic blood pressure is the point at which the pulse sounds become muffled. Some institutions record all three sounds (e.g., 108/70/50).

Situation 3
A low-pitched sound immediately following S_2 and heard best at the apex is an S_3. If it's caused by ventricular abnormality, it's called a ventricular gallop; but it's frequently heard in children and young adults with normal cardiac function. S_3 is caused by the vibrations in the ventricles rapidly filling with blood. Record this finding in your notes. You need not notify the doctor unless there are other signs of cardiac disease.

Situation 4
This pattern is termed sinus arrhythmia. During inspiration a greater volume of blood is drawn into the pulmonary vessels, decreasing the flow of pulmonary blood into the left atrium and left ventricle. The heart rate automatically increases to make up for the lower cardiac output. During expiration, when the cardiac output is higher, the heart rate slows. Sinus arrhythmia is normal in both children and adults.

Situation 5
An S_3 on auscultation.

Situation 6
Aortic stenosis.

Situation 7
Polycythemia.

Situation 8
The mechanism is different in the two kinds of cardiac anomalies. In acyanotic defects (VSD, ASD, PDA, and coarctation of the aorta), the left-to-right shunt produces pulmonary system overload and interstitial edema. The edema, a good culture medium for bacteria, predisposes the child to frequent respiratory in-

fections. In cyanotic defects (tetralogy of Fallot and transposition of the great vessels), some or all of the circulating blood bypasses the lung's cleansing filtration. This predisposes to respiratory complications.

Situation 9
Low cardiac output.

Situation 10
Start oxygen. The PVCs may be caused by myocardial ischemia. Document the arrhythmia with EKG strips and take a 12-lead EKG to make sure that they're ventricular ectopics. Once you've established this diagnosis, give antiarrhythmic medication and notify a doctor immediately. See that a serum potassium level is drawn — Paul may have hypokalemia. The PVCs may also be related to the surgical procedure.

ANSWERS TO SKILLCHECK 2 (page 151)

Situation 1
Hypertension makes the heart work harder as a result of constricted peripheral circulation.

Situation 2
Myocardial nerve endings transmit pain to the upper thoracic posterior roots.

Situation 3
All of these patients may get a pulmonary embolus, but the last patient is most at risk statistically because of his long immobilization. An immobile patient's blood flow is decreased 50% with pooling in dependent body areas from generalized vasodilation. Decreased blood flow and pooling are major causes of thrombus formation.

Situation 4
Several complications could explain Martha's symptoms: myocardial infarction, pericarditis, pneumonia, bronchitis, an episode of supraventricular tachycardia (although this does not explain her elevated temperature), or pulmonary embolus. Any one of these is possible. But Martha's immobilization for over 3 weeks makes pulmonary embolus or pneumonia the most likely. A lung scan would differentiate between them.

Elevate the head of the bed to 45° and administer oxygen by mask or nasal cannula immediately. Notify her doctor. While awaiting orders, start an I.V. (in case shock develops and for the possible administration of anticoagulant medication and digitalis) and do an EKG. Reassure the patient and do not leave her alone.

Situation 5
John's optic fundi show an advanced stage of malignant hypertension. The prognosis is grave and his condition requires vigorous medical management.

Situation 6
CPK-MB.

Situation 7
S-T depression.

Situation 8
Inderal reduces myocardial oxygen consumption by decreasing heart rate and contractility.

Situation 9
Nausea and vomiting are common vagal responses to AMI pain and may also be side effects of morphine. Usually these symptoms end spontaneously. Remember, however, that persistent vomiting can cause potassium depletion (lost in the gastric contents). Hypokalemia can cause arrhythmias. Since the AMI patient is already at risk for life-threatening arrhythmias, make sure serum potassium levels are within normal limits if a patient has been vomiting. He may need a potassium supplement.

Situation 10
You hear 3 heart sounds in the following order: S_4, S_1, S_2. S_4 (atrial gallop) occurs at the end of ventricular diastole when the atria contract and send a bolus of blood into an already blood-filled ventricle. If the left ventricle is stiff (noncompliant) because of the infarction, the vibrations from the blood entering the ventricle are transmitted to the chest wall as a low-pitched sound. Almost all AMI patients have S_4 during the first couple of days and you should not be alarmed. You should, however, chart it in your nursing notes.

Situation 11
All three of the cardiac enzymes (SGOT, LDH, and CPK) occur in skeletal muscle, as well as in the myocardium. Give all pain medication intravenously instead of intramuscularly to avoid raising these.

Situation 12
John's decreased level of consciousness and vital signs all point to cardiac tamponade. Suspect rupture of the heart (a fatal complication of AMI). This is an

extreme emergency. Even with quick intervention, the patient's prognosis is very poor.

ANSWERS TO SKILLCHECK 3 (page 169)

Situation 1
Most likely, Mr. Loger has arterial insufficiency. In venous insufficiency, leg pain usually gets better with walking, not worse; in osteoarthritis or neuropathy, the pain usually persists, even after rest. Mr. Loger has the classical symptoms of arterial insufficiency: His leg pain comes on exertion and goes away within a few minutes upon resting.

Situation 2
Ask Mr. Loger to lie on his back while you raise his legs about 2 feet above the bed or examining table for about 1 minute. Pallor in the legs supports a diagnosis of arterial insufficiency.

Situation 3
Having had a job that required prolonged standing and walking for a number of years supports a diagnosis of primary or superficial varicosities. Phlebography is used to distinguish between primary and secondary (deep thrombophlebitis) varicosities.

Situation 4
Leg cramps at night, nodules or ropelike formations in the legs and swollen calves.

Situation 5
Walking relieves venous symptoms.

Situation 6
Both ischemic and venous stasis are causes of leg ulcers.

Situation 7
Palpation: 80% of abdominal aneurysms are palpable.

Situation 8
Abdominal aneurysms usually occur in persons over 60.

Situation 9
In 95% of cases, arterial aneurysms result from atherosclerosis. Other causes: trauma, congenital defect, syphilis, cystic medionecrosis, or inflammation.

Situation 10
False. A fusiform aneurysm is one that bulges out on both sides of an affected vessel. When all vessel layers rupture, this is called a false aneurysm.

APPENDICES

CARDIAC REHABILITATION PLAN
FOR GRADUATED ACTIVITY AND EXERCISE

IN HOSPITAL	EXERCISE	ACTIVITY
Day 2	Passive range of motion (ROM) to all extremities in bed; active plantar extension and dorsiflexion	Bedside commode; feed self; groom self
Days 3-4	Active ROM (up to 10X)	Bathe self under supervision
Days 5-7	Minimal resistance to active ROM 10X each	Walk back and forth in room twice q.i.d.
Days 8-9	Moderate resistance to active ROM 10X each	Stand at sink to shave; walk to bathroom under observation p.r.n.
Day 10	Add: Exercise: 3 arm and shoulder motions, 5 lateral bends and knee raises, and 5 side leg raises	Bathe in tub or shower; walk in hall b.i.d.
Days 11-12	Add: Sitting on flat bed, touch toes, and twist trunk twice.	Sit up most of day; walk length of hall b.i.d.
Days 13-14	Add: 3 standing half knee bends	Walk at will including up and down one flight of stairs

The above regimen is done under the direct supervision of the cardiac rehabilitation team. The activities should terminate whenever the pulse rate exceeds 115 BPM or ectopic beats occur.

SOME HEART-SAVING ADVICE FOR PATIENTS AFTER DISCHARGE

Eat 4 small meals a day; eat them slowly.

Avoid situations, people, and conditions that make you tense, upset, or angry.

Plan your activities to allow your heart to rest:
—Plan and spread out your work to avoid overload and allow rest between chores.
—If you get tired, no matter what you are doing, stop and rest for 15 to 20 minutes. Don't push yourself to finish mowing the grass, or watch the last 30 minutes of that television show.
—Try not to hurry.
—Plan a 30-minute rest period twice a day.
—Get 6 to 8 hours sleep each night.
—Avoid working with arms above shoulder level. Don't wash windows or hang clothes on the line.

During the first weeks at home continue to be as active as you were on the last day in the hospital. You can do the following things: Get up and get dressed every day.

Walk daily, as much as you were walking in the hospital. You may walk outside when the weather is nice but walk on level ground. Avoid steps and hills. Avoid walking against the wind because your heart works harder and beats faster then. In the winter, walk during the warmest part of the day; in the summer, walk in the morning or evening when it is cool. Walk after a rest period, or when you are not tired. If you have chest discomfort or shortness of breath, stop and sit down on the steps or curb, take nitroglycerin if you have some, and wait until you feel OK again. Tell your doctor about this pain when you see him.

Climb stairs only once a day. You may need to take only a few steps at a time and stop and rest. Avoid doing anything which tenses your body, such as:
● straining when having a bowel movement (ask your doctor about a laxative)
● lifting anything heavy — children, groceries, or suitcases
● pushing or pulling anything heavy
● trying to open a stuck window or unscrew a stuck jar lid.

During later weeks home
Ask your doctor when you may:
● drive the car
● return to work
● go fishing
● go to the movies
● go to a ball game
● roll up your hair.

You may cut the lawn with a self-propelled mower or riding mower. Do this activity with care and in cool weather.

When your doctor says you may work, try to arrange to go back part time at first and then slowly increase your working time.

You may have other questions about your activities, diet, medication, or illness. If you do, feel free to ask your doctor.

General advice
If you develop pain, numbness, or shortness of breath, stop what you are doing, take your nitroglycerin, and rest for several minutes. When the discomfort disappears, continue what you were doing at a slower rate.

Follow your fat-controlled diet. It is an important part of the doctor's plan to help reduce your blood cholesterol.

Continue the physical therapy exercises started in the hospital until you return to normal activity. Do these exercises twice daily.

After a meal, your heart is already working to digest your food. Therefore, rest for an hour after eating before doing any heavy exercise.

Stop smoking. Smoking cigarettes increases your chance of having another heart attack.

If your doctor says you may have liquor, drink in moderation.

Check with your doctor before you take a long trip. As you travel, stop every two hours and walk around to prevent clots from forming in your lower legs. Also, check with your doctor before going to the mountains or to a hot, humid place. Airplane trips are usually permitted one month after your discharge.

As with other activities you should not have sex if:
● you are tired — take a 30-minute nap first
● you have just eaten a heavy meal
● you have been drinking
● you are angry with your mate
● the temperature of the room is uncomfortably warm or cool.

If you begin to have chest discomfort, STOP. The next time, try taking nitroglycerin beforehand. Remember, it's normal for your heart to beat faster and your breathing to speed up during sexual activity. Your heart beat and breathing should slow down and return to normal shortly afterward.

Notify your doctor immediately whenever you have:
● heavy pressure or squeezing pain in the chest which may spread to the shoulder, arm, neck, or jaw and is not relieved in 15 minutes by resting and/or nitroglycerin
● increased shortness of breath
● unusual tiredness
● swelling of feet and ankles
● fainting
● very slow or rapid heart rate.

SOME CARDIOVASCULAR DRUGS

DRUG	USE, ROUTE, AND DOSAGE	SIDE EFFECTS	NURSING TIPS
atropine sulfate◊	Anticholinergic, (for bradycardia) I.V. bolus 0.5 mg, may repeat	Therapeutic dosages: dry mouth, cycloplegia, mydriasis. Large dosages: hyperpyrexia, urinary retention, confusion, and hallucinations.	• When protocol allows, give to patients with bradycardia (rate < 50 BPM) who have hypotension, syncope, and dyspnea.
clonidine hydrochloride Catapres	Antihypertensive P.O.: initial dose 0.1 mg b.i.d. increase by 0.1-0.2 mg per day until desired response obtained; usual maintenance dose is 0.2-0.8 mg daily in divided doses	Dry mouth, drowsiness, sedation, constipation, dizziness, headache, fatigue.	• Don't discontinue abruptly • Warn patient about sedative effect • Patient should not drink alcohol or take sedatives with this drug • Periodic eye exams are necessary because of potential ocular toxicity (not yet shown in human studies).
calcium chloride◊	Cardiac stimulant I.V. bolus, intracardiac 1 g (10 ml of a 10% sol), may repeat	Cardiac arrhythmia (in digitalized patients), venous irritation, vasodilation, hypotension, bradycardia, syncope, cardiac arrest.	• Very irritating; take extreme care to avoid extravasation when giving I.V. • Avoid using in digitalized patients; may cause fatal arrhythmia.
dopamine hydrochloride Intropin◊	Adrenergic; inotropic agent I.V. infusion 5 mcg/kg/min up to 20-50 mcg/kg/min	Ectopic beats, tachycardia, angina, palpitation, vasoconstriction, hypotension, dyspnea, nausea and vomiting, headache.	• Do not add to alkaline solutions, e.g. sodium bicarbonate • Monitor EKG for ventricular arrhythmias • Check urine output q 30 min • Rate of infusion is adjusted according to cardiac output, peripheral perfusion, urine output, and pulmonary and arterial pressures, so monitor all these parameters closely • Must be diluted to 250-500 ml volume before using.
disopyramide phosphate Norpace Rhythmodan◊◊	Antiarrhythmic P.O.: loading dose — 300 mg then 100-150 mg q6h	Dry mouth, eyes, nose, throat, urinary hesitancy or retention, urinary frequency or urgency, GI distress, constipation, blurred vision, weight gain (edema), headache, generalized fatigue and weakness, dizziness, rash, nervousness, hypotension, shortness of breath, chest pain, syncope.	• Don't give to patients in cardiogenic shock, 2nd or 3rd degree A-V block • Give cautiously to patients with renal or liver disease • If hypotension or heart failure occurs, notify the doctor immediately.

◊ Also available in Canada.
◊◊ Available in Canada only.

SOME CARDIOVASCULAR DRUGS

DRUG	USE, ROUTE, AND DOSAGE	SIDE EFFECTS	NURSING TIPS
epinephrine hydrochloride Adrenalin◇	Adrenergic, cardiac stimulant I.V. bolus, intracardiac 0.5-1 mg (5-10 ml of 1:10,000 sol); may repeat	Fear, anxiety, headache, tremor, dizziness, disorientation, nausea and vomiting, sweating, pallor, respiratory difficulty and apnea, palpitation, tachycardia, angina, ventricular arrhythmias.	• Watch for ventricular decompensation and pulmonary edema due to peripheral vasoconstriction • Stop if headache, chest pain, nausea, or hypotension occur • I.V. injection of 1:1000 sol leads to hypertension, sub-arachnoid hemorrhage and hemiplegia
guanethidine sulfate Ismelin◇	Antihypertensive P.O.: 25-50 mg daily; up to 300 mg daily in severe hypertension	Orthostatic hypotension, dizziness, weakness, lassitude, bradycardia, nasal congestion, diarrhea, inhibition of ejaculation, edema.	• Use cautiously in patients with renal disease (lowered BP may further compromise renal function) • Don't give to patients with severe cardiac failure; blocks the body's natural adrenergic compensatory mechanism
hydralazine hydrochloride Apresoline◇ Rolazine	Antihypertensive P.O.: Initial dose 10 mg q.i.d. for 4 days, then 25 mg q.i.d. for 3 days, then 50 mg q.i.d. thereafter. Maintenance: lowest effective dose I.V., I.M.: 20-40 mg repeated as necessary	Headache, palpitations, GI disturbance, tachycardia, angina, flushing, peripheral neuritis, edema, anxiety, lupus-like syndrome.	• Don't discontinue abruptly • Watch for signs of myo-cardial ischemia: angina, EKG changes • Use cautiously in patients with suspected coronary artery disease.
isoproterenol hydrochloride Isuprel◇	Adrenergic, cardiac stimulant I.V. bolus, intracardiac 0.02 mg; I.V. infusion of 1 mg/500 ml D₅W titrated to heart rate and blood pressure	Arrhythmias, palpitation, tachycardia, headache, flushing, dizziness, sweating, tremors.	• Slow or stop infusion if heart rate exceeds rate of 110/min • Discontinue if ventricular arrhythmia occurs • Have defibrillator at bedside • Measure urine output and B.P. every 15 min • Do not use concurrently with epinephrine, may cause serious arrhythmias.
levarterenol bitartrate Levophed◇	Adrenergic, vasopressor I.V. infusion 8-16 mg (2-4 amps) in 500 ml D₅W titrated to blood pressure	Intense sweating, vomiting, severe hypertension, head-ache, weakness, dizziness, tremor, pallor, respiratory difficulty, precordial pain, cardiac arrhythmias, tissue necrosis and sloughing from extravasation of injection.	• Check infusion site frequently to avoid extravasation • Should extravasation occur, stop infusion, flush the area immediately with 15 ml of saline and 10 ml of phentolamine to avoid sloughing of tissue • Guanethidine and methyldopa increase levarterenol's effect.

◇ Also available in Canada.
◇◇ Available in Canada only.

SOME CARDIOVASCULAR DRUGS

DRUG	USE, ROUTE, AND DOSAGE	SIDE EFFECTS	NURSING TIPS
lidocaine hydrochloride Xylocaine◇	Ventricular antiarrhythmic I.V. bolus 100 mg followed by I.V. infusion 1-2 g/500 ml D₅W at 2-4 mg/min	Hypotension, cardiovascular collapse, bradycardia, convulsions, respiratory depression, visual disturbances, slurred speech. Severe reactions may be preceded by somnolence and paresthesia.	● Give cautiously to patients with Stokes-Adam syndrome, liver disease or CHF — may cause toxicity ● If CNS side effects occur, stop the infusion immediately, give O₂, and call the doctor.
metaraminol bitartrate Aramine◇	Adrenergic, vasopressor I.V. 15-100 mg/500 ml D₅/NSS I.M. 2-10 mg	Anxiety, tremor, faintness, headache, dizziness, precordial pain, respiratory difficulty, flushing, pallor, sweating, nausea.	● Monitor vital signs q 30 min ● MAO inhibitors potentiate its pressor effect ● Guanethedine — metaraminol interaction may cause hypertensive crisis.
methyldopa Aldomet◇	Antihypertensive P.O.: Initial dose 250 mg b.i.d. or t.i.d. for 2 days, then increase or decrease dose every 2 days until desired effect obtained. Maintenance: 500 mg-3 g daily in 2-4 doses. I.V. infusion: 250-500 mg (maximum dose 1 g) in 100 ml D₅W over 30-60 min q6h (dose titrated according to BP)	Sedation, headache, and weakness (all transient); orthostatic hypotension, edema, GI distress, liver function test abnormalities, positive Coombs' test, drug fever, rash, impotence, dry mouth, nasal stuffiness, lactation.	● Use cautiously in patients with liver disease ● Warn patients about sedative effect ● Baseline blood count recommended at start and periodically during therapy.
nitroprusside sodium Nipride◇	Vasodilator, antihypertensive I.V. 0.5-10 mcg/kg/min. continuous I.V. infusion. Use only D₅W for dilution; to make solution containing 100 mcg/ml dilute 50 mg nitroprusside in 500 ml D₅W	GI disturbance, increased perspiration, headache, restlessness, apprehension, muscle twitching, retrosternal discomfort, palpitations, dizziness, hypotension, irritation at infusion site.	● Protect container and tubing from light ● Prepare fresh infusion every 4 hours ● Use infusion pump ● Avoid extravasation ● Monitor vital signs q 5 min while the infusion is being started, then q 15 min.
prazosin hydrochloride Minipress◇	Antihypertensive P.O.: Initial dose 1 mg t.i.d. Maintenance: 3-20 mg daily in divided doses (a few patients may require up to 40 mg daily)	Severe syncope with loss of consciousness if initial dose greater than 1 mg; headache, drowsiness, weakness, palpitations, GI disturbance, edema, dry mouth, dizziness.	● Observe closely for syncopal episodes after initial dose and each dosage increase. Such episodes usually occur within 60-90 min after dose.
procainamide hydrochloride Procainamide◇ Pronestyl◇	Ventricular antiarrhythmic P.O.: 250-500 mg q3-4h I.M.: 0.5-1 g q6h until patient can take drug P.O. I.V.: 100 mg q5 min. (at rate of 20-50 mg/min) up to max. loading dose of 1g or until arrhythmia suppressed. Drip of 1-4 mg/min may be used after loading dose.	Hypotension and serious disturbances of cardiac rhythm due to Q-T prolongation with I.M. or I.V. routes: GI disturbances, urticaria, pruritus, fever, chills, weakness, depression, psychosis, lupus-like syndrome and positive ANA test (during prolonged therapy), agranulocytosis.	● Watch for cardiac arrhythmias, atrial fibrillation and ventricular tachycardia after I.V. administration ● Tell patient to report any sore throat or sores in mouth, unexplained fever or upper respiratory tract infection ● Use I.V. route only for emergencies.

◇ Also available in Canada.
◇◇ Available in Canada only.

SOME CARDIOVASCULAR DRUGS

DRUG	USE, ROUTE, AND DOSAGE	SIDE EFFECTS	NURSING TIPS
propranolol hydrochloride Inderal	Antihypertensive, antianginal, antiarrhythmic P.O.: Hypertension, 80-640 mg daily in divided doses; angina and arrhythmias — 10-40 mg q.i.d. I.V.: 1-3 mg	Bradycardia, CHF, intensification of A-V block, hypotension, light-headedness, visual disturbances, GI distress, bronchospasm, exacerbation of angina and MI may follow abrupt withdrawal of drug, mental disturbances ranging from disorientation to catatonia.	• Do not discontinue abruptly • Note small I.V. dose compared to P.O. dose • Use I.V. route only for life-threatening arrhythmias • May mask signs of hypoglycemia in diabetic patients.
quinidine Quinidine sulfate◇ Quiniglute Dura-Tabs◇ Cardioquin◇ Biquin Durules◇◇ Quinate◇◇ Quinidine gluconate	Atrial and ventricular antiarrhythmic P.O.: *Test dose*, 200 mg to determine idiosyncrasy, then 200-300 mg q4-6h I.M.: Initial dose 300-400 mg, then 200 mg q2h, times four (for acute tachycardia) I.V. Infusion: Dilute 800 mg in 50 ml D₅W. Administer at rate of 16 mg/min or 1 ml/min. Dose of less than 300 mg usually terminates arrhythmia.	Tinnitus, headache, disturbed vision, cardiac asystole, ventricular arrhythmias, widening of QRS complex, paradoxical tachycardia, GI disturbance, vertigo, excitement, confusion, cutaneous flushing with intense pruritus, hypersensitivity reaction, fever.	• Give test dose (200 mg) to determine idiosyncrasy; observe patient closely; take vital signs frequently • Give cautiously to patients in incomplete A-V block (may cause complete A-V block) • Widening of QRS complex 50% is sign of quinidine cardiotoxicity. Stop drug immediately.
reserpine Reserpine Serpasil◇ Reserpanca◇◇ NEO-Serp◇◇	Antihypertensive P.O.: Initial dose, 0.5 mg daily for 1-2 weeks. Maintenance, 0.1-0.25 mg daily. I.M.: (hypertensive crisis) initial dose 0.5-1.0 mg, then 2-4 mg q3h until desired response	Depression, GI disturbances including hypersecretion, angina-like symptoms, arrhythmias, drowsiness, nervousness, anxiety, nightmares, dull sensorium, deafness, nasal congestion, pruritus, rash, dry mouth, dizziness, headache, impotence, dysuria, myalgias, edema.	• Use cautiously in patients with renal disease (lowered BP may further compromise renal function) • Avoid in patients with history of mental depression • Watch closely for signs of developing despondency • Contraindicated in patients with ulcer disease or ulcerative colitis.
sodium bicarbonate*	To prevent acidosis I.V. bolus 1 mEq/kg, repeat in 10 min. if necessary. Further doses based on blood gas analysis. If ABGs unavailable, use 0.5 mEq/kg every 10 min during resuscitation.	Metabolic alkalosis.	• Incompatible with calcium solutions • A 4.2% solution, slow administration preferred for children under 2 • Watch for signs of alkalosis: nausea, vomiting, diarrhea, respirations slow and shallow, confusion, irritability, twitching.

◇Available in Canada
◇◇Available in Canada only

GLOSSARY

acidosis — a condition in which excessive hydrogen ions (pH) are present in body fluids due to loss of base or retention of noncarbonic acids.

akinesis — temporary paralysis or failure of part of the cardiac muscle to contract during systole.

alkalosis — opposite of acidosis, occurs with decreased hydrogen ion (pH) concentration in body fluids due to loss of acid or retention of base.

amniotic fluid embolism — a fatal condition caused by an embolus of amniotic fluid, vernix, or meconium entering the pulmonary circulation.

amyloid — a waxy, translucent, insoluble glycoprotein; occurs in many conditions and leaves tissues waxy and nonfunctional.

anasarca — generalized massive edema.

aneurysm — a sac formed by the bulging wall of an artery or vein.

angina pectoris — chest pain due to insufficient delivery of oxygen to the myocardium. Status anginosus — angina occurring at rest and resistant to treatment.

angiogram — visualization of a blood vessel due to injection of a contrast medium.

angiotensin — a vasoconstrictor found in blood.

anoxia — oxygen deficiency in body tissue due to reduced blood flow or other causes resulting in tissue injury or death.

anticholinergic — an effect that blocks impulse transmission across the parasympathetic ganglia; a substance that blocks the effects of acetycholine.

apnea — cessation of respirations.

arrhythmia — any disturbance in rate, rhythm, or conduction of the heart.

arteriography — visualization of an artery/arteries after injection of a radiopaque material into the blood stream.

arteriosclerosis — a group of diseases which result in thickening and loss of elasticity of arterial walls.

ascites — abnormal accumulation of fluid in the abdominal cavity.

asynchronism — disturbance of the time factor in the cardiac contraction sequence.

asyneresis — localized contraction of part of the heart muscle that is uniform in length but lacks force.

atelectasis — collapse of all or part of a lung.

atherosclerosis — narrowing of the lumen of arterial walls via the accumulation of fatty plaques.

atria — the collecting chambers for blood brought into the heart from the venae cavae and from the lungs.

atrioventricular (AV) node — a group of specialized cardiac muscle fibers located in the floor of the right atrium that carry electrical impulses from the atria to the bundle of His.

autoimmune — immunologic action against the body's own tissue.

bigeminal rhythm — beats that occur in pairs — one normal, one premature (atrial or ventricular).

bradycardia — abnormal slowness of heart rate; usually fewer than 60 beats per minute.

Buerger's disease — a chronic recurring inflammatory disease affecting the arteries and veins especially in the legs. Also known as thromboangiitis obliterans.

bundle of His — group of specialized muscle fibers in the interventricular septum of the heart; conveys electrical impulses from the AV node to the Purkinje fibers to stimulate ventricular contraction.

cardiac angiography — X-ray examination of the coronary arteries after a radiopaque dye has been injected into them.

cardiac catheterization — a diagnostic test in which a catheter is introduced into a blood vessel and maneuvered into the heart. The purpose of this procedure is to obtain blood samples from the heart, detect abnormalities, and determine intracardiac pressure.

cardiac cycle — one heartbeat; time required for heart to complete filling (diastole) and emptying (systole) — usually 8/10 of a second.

cardiac output — force and volume of blood pumped out of the heart per minute.

cardiomegaly — enlarged heart muscle. Chambers generally remain normal size with excess tissue accumulation.

cardiomyopathy — general term meaning disease of the heart muscle, usually of unknown etiology.

cardioversion — restoration of rapid, abnormal rates and/or rhythms to normal sinus rhythm by drug or electrical countershock.

carotid artery — main artery in the neck, consists of right and left branches that lie on either side of the larynx.

carotid sinus — a dilated portion of the common carotid artery, just above the bifurcation of the two main branches, containing a rich supply of nerve endings from the sinus branch of the vagus nerve.

central venous pressure (CVP) — the pressure exerted by the blood in the venae cavae and right atrium.

Chagas' disease — a form of trypanosomiasis prevalent in Central and South America. Also called Chagas-Cruz disease, it is transmitted by the reduviid bug.

Cheyne-Stokes respiration — abnormal pattern characterized by slow, shallow breathing that increases in depth and rapidity until it reaches an apex from which it decreases gradually and ceases altogether for a short period; cycle then resumes.

claudication — pain in legs during walking, due to inadequate blood supply or venous drainage. Pain subsides with rest.

clubbing — occurs with congenital heart disease and chronic pulmonary disease when the ends of the fingers or toes become swollen and soft and take on a rounded appearance.

coarctation — narrowing or constriction of a vessel; of aorta: causes increased cardiac activity, hypertension in the arms and hypotension in the legs.

collateral — alternate vascular route formed when original becomes obstructed or reduced.

colloid — a substance which, when in solution, remains suspended, neither dissolving nor settling.

congenital defect — malformation of the heart or one of its major blood vessels present at birth.

coronary — the circulatory system of the heart; a nerve or blood vessel that encircles the heart.

coronary arteries — two arteries arising from the aorta that supply the heart muscle with blood.

cor pulmonale — a serious condition in which increased pressure within the pulmonary artery results in right ventricular heart failure.

coronary occlusion — an obstruction or narrowing of one of the coronary arteries that inhibits the flow of blood to some part of the heart muscle.

creatine phosphokinase (CPK) — an enzyme found in the skeletal muscles, heart, and brain that is released by inflammatory processes.

creatinine — a normal, alkaline, nonprotein end product of metabolism present in the blood and urine.

crystalloid — a substance capable of forming crystals and of passing through a semi-permeable membrane.

cyanosis — a bluish-gray discoloration of the skin resulting from a deficiency of oxygen and an excess of carbon dioxide in the blood.

defibrillator — delivers electrical impulses to the heart causing temporary cessation of cardiac activity, allowing time for the SA node to take over.

deMusset's sign — rhythmic shaking of the head due to pulsations of the carotid arteries, a sign of aortic insufficiency.

depolarization — equalization of ions on both sides of cell membrane with loss of electrical charge or polarity.

diaphoresis — excessive perspiration.

diastole — relaxation phase of cardiac cycle when ventricles are filling; between contractions.

Dressler's syndrome — postmyocardial infarction syndrome. A group of symptoms thought to result from antigen-antibody reaction and difficult to distinguish from extension or recurrence of an infarction.

dyskinesis — difficult or impaired expansion of part of the ventricular wall during systole.

dyspnea — difficult or labored breathing.

echocardiography — ultrasonic waves directed through the chest wall transmitting and recording the position and motion of the heart and valves.

ectopic focus — in cardiology, a source of cardiac stimulus other than the SA node; usually caused by some irritation of the myocardium.

edema — excessive accumulation of fluid in body tissues.

electrophoresis — a laboratory method used to analyze the plasma's protein content.

embolus — undissolved matter in the bloodstream; a traveling thrombus.

endocardium — the endothelial lining of the heart.

epicardium — outer covering of the heart; also called the visceral pericardium.

escape. *See ventricular.*

extrasystole — a premature contraction of the heart.

fibrillation — abnormal, rapid, chaotic arrhythmia of either atria or ventricles which prevents efficient myocardial contractility.

gallop rhythm — the occurrence of three or four extra heart sounds during diastole.

HDL — high density lipoproteins — high levels in the blood serum indicate a decreased risk of coronary heart disease.

heart block — impaired impulse conduction of the heart; can occur any place in the heart; usually applied to atrioventricular heart block.

hematocrit — volume percentage of erythrocytes in whole blood.

hemodynamics — the movements and forces that maintain circulation.

hemoglobin — that part of the red blood cells that carries oxygen.

hemothorax — an accumulation of blood in the pleural cavity.

histamine — an amine, present in all body tissue; causes dilation of capillaries, increased gastric secretion, and constriction of bronchial smooth muscles.

holosystolic — refers to the entire systolic phase of the cardiac cycle.

Holter monitor — ambulatory electrocardiography; useful in diagnosing arrhythmias and causes of CNS symptoms such as dizziness, syncope, and pain.

hyperkalemia — excessive accumulation of potassium in the blood.

hyperlipidemia — abnormally high levels of lipids (fats) in the blood.

hyperpnea — a detectable increase in respiratory rate, above that normally seen in resting individuals.

hypertrophy — increased size of an organ or structure due to functional activity; not an increase in cells or tissue.

hypovolemia — abnormal decrease in blood volume.

ischemia — localized deficiency of blood caused by constriction or obstruction of the blood vessel to that area.

isoelectric — the base line in an electrocardiogram.

millivolt — one-thousandth of a volt.

monitor — to watch continuously, observing and recording vital signs and other pertinent data; an apparatus used to observe and record physiological signs, e.g. EKG, Holter monitor, etc.

mural — occurring in or referring to the wall of an organ or part. (Example: Mural thrombus occurs on the interior wall of the heart.)

murmur — a sound heard upon auscultation of the heart. It is produced by vibrations caused by the movement of the blood in the heart and large vessels during systole or diastole.

muscular dystrophy — a group of related muscle diseases characterized by wasting away and atrophy of the muscles.

myocardial catecholamines — group of neurohormones having an adrenergic effect on the heart.

myocardial infarction — tissue necrosis caused by myocardial ischemia.

myocardial insufficiency — weakening of the heart muscle that reduces the force whereby blood is ejected from the heart.

myocardial ischemia — a condition resulting from blood and oxygen starvation of the heart muscle.

myocardium — heart muscle.

myxoma, atrial — a benign gelatinous growth composed of primitive, mucous connective tissue.

necrosis — tissue death.

nephrosclerosis — a hardening of the kidney due to renovascular disease.

neurohormones — hormones that stimulate neural responses.

nocturia — unusually frequent urination occurring at night.

orthopnea — difficulty breathing except in an upright position.

pacemaker — the SA node, so called because it initiates the electrical impulses that set the rhythm of cardiac contractions. An artificial pacemaker: an electrical device to pace cardiac rhythm; used particularly when a patient has a heart block.

palpitations — awareness of excessively rapid, fluttering heartbeats; may produce a high degree of anxiety.

papilledema — swelling of the optic disk; usually associated with intracranial pressure.

paradoxical pulse — fades away on inspiration and is weak on expiration due to changed intrathoracic pressures.

paroxysmal atrial tachycardia (PAT) — an arrhythmia characterized by the sudden onset of rapid, regular heartbeats in excess of 150-250 beats per minute.

PCO₂ — the tension exerted by carbon dioxide in arterial blood.

perfusion — injecting or pouring fluid over or through an organ.

pericardiocentesis — puncture of the sac around the heart for the purpose of withdrawing fluid.

pericardium — a fibroserous, fluid-filled sac surrounding the heart and the origins of the great vessels; composed of two layers, the visceral and the parietal.

peripheral vascular resistance — the force opposing the flow of blood through the vessels; depends on the size of the vessel and viscosity of fluid it contains.

petechiae — small, purplish, nonraised spots on the surface of the skin caused by intradermal or submucous hemorrhage.

pH — hydrogen ion concentration; denotes acidity or alkalinity of a solution; a pH over 7 means a solution is alkaline; under 7, means acid.

pheochromocytoma — a tumor of the adrenal medulla that causes hypertension by overproducing adrenal hormones.

phlebothrombosis — clotting in a vein unassociated with inflammation of the vessel walls.

phonocardiography — sounds of heart action recorded graphically on paper.

plaque — an accumulation of fatty material within the arterial intima.

pleura — moist lining of the chest wall that encloses the pleural cavity.

pneumothorax — air or gas in the pleural cavity that causes collapse of all or part of a lung.

polymyositis — inflammation of many muscles occurring simultaneously.

precordial — pertaining to that region over the heart and stomach, the epigastrium, and lower part of the thorax.

premature ventricular contraction (PVC) — the most common ventricular arrhythmia, it occurs during diastole and originates from a focus somewhere in the ventricle. It may be normal or the result of irritation, ischemia, or drug therapy.

prophylactic — a chemical or physical agent used to ward off disease.

prostaglandins — first identified in seminal fluid, they are now known to be present in cells all over the body. Derivatives of fatty cells, they appear to alter certain chemical reactions in the body.

pulmonary wedge pressure (PWP) — measures left atrial pressure and left ventricular end diastolic pressure (LVEDP) by means of a bulb-tipped catheter wedged in a small branch of the pulmonary artery; the most accurate means of predicting incipient heart failure.

pulse deficit — difference between apical and radial pulses when taken simultaneously.

pulsus alternans — strong beats alternating with weak beats while heart rhythm remains uninterrupted.

pulsus bisferiens — two arterial pulsations of almost equal strength per one heartbeat.

Purkinje fibers — located in the ventricles, they constitute an important part of the impulse-conduction system of the heart.

rales — abnormal respiratory sound heard on auscultation.

Raynaud's phenomenon — arterial spasms of the extremities precipitated by cold. They cause blanching, cold, and numbness followed by redness, warmth, and tingling.

refractory — resistant to treatment.

repolarization — return to resting potential or polarity in the cell membrane.

retinopathy — generally any noninflammatory disease of the retina.

retractions — the shortening of a muscle fiber in preparation for release of energy.

rheumatic heart disease — permanent damage to the heart, usually valvular, caused by recurrent attacks of rheumatic fever.

sarcoidosis — a chronic, progressive, generalized disorder that may affect any part of the body but especially lymph tissue; characterized by the presence of epithelioid cell tubercles that gradually change to fibrous tissue.

septum — a wall or partition dividing an organ or body part.

serum glutamic oxaloacetic transaminase (SGOT) — an enzyme present in cardiac cells which escapes into the bloodstream upon tissue death and can be measured to assess damage.

sick sinus syndrome — alternating tachy- and brady-arrhythmia that appears in chronic ischemic heart disease when the SA node cannot respond correctly.

sino-atrial (SA) node — a small collection of neuromuscular tissue located near the junction of the superior vena cava and right atrium which normally serves as the cardiac pacemaker.

stenosis — a narrowing or constricting of an opening.

Stokes-Adams syndrome — sudden attacks of unconsciousness, sometimes coupled with convulsions, which may accompany heart block or ventricular arrhythmia as a result of low cardiac output.

Swan-Ganz catheter — a flow-directed, balloon-tipped catheter inserted in a central venous position and advanced to the pulmonary artery; used to monitor pulmonary capillary or wedge pressure.

sympatholytics — agents that block the transmission of impulses from the adrenergic postganglionic fibers to effector organs or tissues inhibiting smooth-muscle contraction and glandular secretion.

synchronous — occurring simultaneously.

syndrome — a group of symptoms that form a specific disease pattern.

systole — the contraction phase of the heart muscle that forces blood from the ventricles into the pulmonary artery and aorta.

tachycardia — heart rate usually greater than 100 beats per minute; it may be sinusal, atrial, junctional, or ventricular.

tachypnea — rapid, shallow breathing.

tamponade, cardiac — an accumulation of blood in the pericardial sac; it compresses the heart and inhibits diastolic filling; also called hemopericardium.

tetralogy of Fallot — congenital heart defect due to structural abnormalities. Referred to as blue babies, the cyanosis results from oxygenated blood from the lungs mixing with oxygen-depleted blood from the systemic circulation.

thoracentesis — surgical puncture of the thoracic cavity for the purpose of removing excess fluid.

thrombolytic agents — drugs that dissolve or break up clots.

thrombophlebitis — the development of clots in the presence of inflammatory changes in venous walls.

thrombus — a stationary clot in the circulatory system that frequently obstructs a vessel or cavity.

thrill — a very fine tremor felt on palpation, produced by an irregularity in blood flow due to a vascular or cardiac murmur; also felt on palpation of aneurysm.

thyrotoxicosis — a thyroid disorder, resulting from overproductivity of thyroid gland, characterized by accelerated pulse rate, exopthalmus, increased metabolic rate, and nervous symptoms.

triglycerides — a kind of lipid in the bloodstream; a glycerol bound to fatty acids.

Valsalva's maneuver — bearing down, or forced exhalation effort against a closed glottis, which slows the heart rate.

varices — enlarged, tortuous abnormalities of the veins that may be caused by increased venous pressure and valvular weakness.

vasoconstrictor – *See vasopressor.*

vasodilator — an agent that relaxes (dilates) venous or arterial vessel walls.

vasopressor — an agent that stimulates generalized vasoconstriction, usually increasing blood flow to the body's vital organs.

vena cava — large vessel that returns blood to the heart: The superior drains from head and upper torso; the inferior from the lower extremities and abdominal cavity.

ventricle — a small cavity: the heart's two muscular lower chambers.

ventricular escape — occurs when impulse conduction in the ventricular pacemaker fires before the impulse in the sinoatrial node.

ventriculography — visualization of the ventricles after introduction of a contrast medium.

COMMON CARDIOVASCULAR ABBREVIATIONS

AAA — abdominal aortic aneurysm
ABG — arterial blood gas
AMI — acute myocardial infarction
ASD — atrial septal defect
ASHD — arteriosclerotic heart disease
ASO — arteriosclerosis obliterans
AV — atrioventricular
BPM — beats per minute
CAD — coronary artery disease
CCU — coronary care unit
CHF — congestive heart failure
COU — coronary observation unit
CPK — creatinine phosphokinase
CPR — cardiopulmonary resuscitation
CVA — cerebrovascular accident
CVP — central venous pressure
EKG — electrocardiogram
HDL — high density lipoprotein
IAPB — intra-aortic balloon pump
ICU — intensive care unit
IHSS — idiopathic hypertrophic subaortic stenosis
LAD — left anterior descending coronary artery
LAP — left atrial pressure
LC — left circumflex artery
LCA — left coronary artery
LDH — lactic dehydrogenase
LM — left main
LVEDP — left ventricular end-diastolic pressure
MCL — midclavicular line
PA — pulmonary arterial (line)
PAC — premature atrial contractions
PAP — pulmonary arterial pressure
PAT — paroxysmal atrial tachycardia
PCO_2 — partial pressure of carbon dioxide
PDA — patent ductus arteriosus
PMI — point of maximal impulse
PO_2 — partial pressure of oxygen
PTT — partial thromboplastin time
PVC — premature ventricular contractions
PWP — pulmonary wedge pressure
RCA — right coronary artery
RHD — rheumatic heart disease
SA — sinoatrial
SBE — subacute bacterial endocarditis
SGOT — serum glutamic oxaloacetic transaminase
VSD — ventricular septal defect

INDEX

Page numbers followed by the letter "t" indicate both tabular and marginal material.

A

Abdominal pain, 164
Acute bacterial endocarditis. See *Endocarditis, bacterial.*
Acute myocardial infarction (AMI). See *Myocardial infarction.*
Adult respiratory distress syndrome, 167
Adults, young, 117
Afterload, 105, 107, 108. See also *Blood pressure, systemic.*
Air embolism, 134t
Akinesis, 64, 85t
Alcohol, 128
Aldosterone, 104
Aldosteronism, primary, 72t
American Heart Association on blood pressure, 18, 67, 74
Amniotic fluid emboli, 134t
Amyloidosis, 126
Anemia, 17t, 20, 22
Aneurysms, 22, 165t, 166t, 167t
  abdominal aortic, 163-168, 168t
  postoperative care and, 167-168
  ventricular, 57-58, 90, 103, 111
Angina, 53t, 79-82, 130
Angina pectoris. See *Angina.*
Angiography, 128, 130, 138, 158
Angiotension, 104
Anorexia, 93-94
Antihypertensive drugs, 71-72
Anxiety, 91
Aorta
  coarctation of, 16t, 19, 27t, 30
  dilation of, 18
  ejection click and, 22
  hypertension and, 70, 72t
  intra-aortic balloon pump and, 108
  tetralogy of Fallot and, 30
Aortic regurgitation, 17t, 19t, 54, 123, 123t
Aortic stenosis, 19t, 20, 22
  endocarditis and, 117, 117t

murmurs and, 54
  pulsus bisferiens and, 17t
Aortic valve, 49, 117
Aorto-iliac block, 158
Apical impulse, 48
Arrhythmias, 20, 39, 130
  acute myocardial infarction and, 86, 87t, 89, 91t
  pericardiocentesis and, 114
  surgery and, 36
  Swan-Ganz catheter and, 106t-107t
  ventricular, 106
Arterial insufficiency, 155-159, 162
Arterial ischemia, 164
Arterial occlusion, 79t, 157t, 158
  aneurysm and, 164
  ASO and, 156
Arterial pressure, 105
Arteries, 52t, 108
Arteriography, 64-65, 64t, 108, 111
Arteriosclerosis obliterans (ASO), 155, 159t. See also *Arterial insufficiency.*
  amputations and, 158
  pain and, 156
Ascites, 94
Assessment. See *Patient assessment.*
Assessment, initial, 45
Assessment tests. See *Diagnostic tests.*
Asthma, 17t
Atelectasis, 144
Atherosclerosis, 69, 78t, 84t, 164t
Atresia. See *Ventricular outflow obstruction.*
Atrial fibrillation, 19-20, 130, 132
Atrial flutter, 19
Atrial gallop, 52, 81, 84
Atrial myxomas, 57
Atrial septal defect (ASD), 22, 26t, 28-29
Atrial systole, 54
Atrioventricular block, 142t
Auscultation, 49-54, 51t, 116
  child and, 19-20, 21t

B

Bacteria, 115, 116, 116t
Behavior problems in child, 40
Beriberi, 128
Bigeminy, 20
Biopsy, 130
Blood flow, 24, 28, 94, 137
Blood pressure, 19t, 68, 74
  cardiogenic shock and, 103-104, 105
  coarctation of aorta and, 30
  decreased, 104, 144
  hypertension and, 71-72, 104
  in children, 18, 18t
  in heart, 24, 52t
  pulsus alternans and, 47
  systemic, 84t
Bradyarrhythmias, 142
Bradycardia, 104
Buerger's disease, 161t

C

Caffeine, 73
Cardiac arrest, 39, 108
Cardiac asthma, 98
Cardiac calcifications, 56-57
Cardiac catheterization, 61-66, 63t, 64t, 111, 124
Cardiac chamber dilatation, 57
Cardiac complications, 103-114
Cardiac contractility, 68
Cardiac cycle, 50-54
Cardiac disease. See *Heart disease.*
Cardiac enlargement. See *Cardiomegaly.*
Cardiac enzymes, 61, 88t
Cardiac ischemia, 59
Cardiac massage, 108
Cardiac monitoring, 144
Cardiac output, 36, 68
  atrial septal defect and, 29
  cardiogenic shock and, 105
  cerebral vascular perfusion and, 104
  drugs and, 105, 106-107, 131
  hypoxemia and, 104
Cardiac shunt, 32
Cardiac surgery. See *Surgery.*
Cardiac tamponade, 38, 103. See

also *Tamponade, cardiac.*
electrode perforation and, 144
heart, rupture of, and, 89-90
Cardiogenic shock, 103-106
  intra-aortic balloon pumps and, 107-108
  myocardial infarction and, 89, 103-111
  prevention of, 111
  pulmonary artery pressure and, 104t
  surgery and, 108
Cardiomegaly, 16, 126
Cardiomegaly, idiopathic. See *Cardiomyopathy.*
Cardiomyopathy, 125-132
  alcoholic, 128, 130
  congestive, 127t, 128, 131
  hypertrophic, 127t, 128, 130, 131
  IHSS, 132
  metabolic, 128
  obliterative, 127t, 128
  patients with, problems of, 130t
  postpartum, 128
  restrictive, 127t, 128, 130, 132
  viruses and, 128
Cardiopulmonary resuscitation (CPR), 113t
Cardiothoracic ratio, 56
Cardiovascular disease, 16, 46, 55-66
Cardiovascular examination, 20t
Cardioversion, 132
Carditis, 123
Central venous pressure, 38, 105
Cerebral vascular perfusion, 104, 137
Cerebrovascular accidents, 71
Chagas' disease. See *Protozoas.*
Chest, 18-22
  inspection of, 46-47
  palpation of, 48
Chest pain, 80-82
  acute myocardial infarction and, 83-84
  arteriography and, 65
  electrocardiogram and, 59
  hypertension and, 70
  pericarditis and, 121-122
Chest tubes, 38-39
Children, 15-22, 21t
  endocarditis and, 117
  honesty in dealing with, 35
  hospitalization and, 34, 38t
  myocarditis and, 115
  rheumatic fever and, 123

surgery and, 33-40
tetralogy of Fallot in, 30-32
transposition of great vessels and, 32
Cholesterol, 75, 76, 78, 81t
Circulation, integumentary changes and, 46
Clubbing, of digits, 16, 29t, 46, 46t
Collateral circulation, 158-159
Congenital heart defects. See *Heart defects, congenital.*
Congestive heart disease. See *Cardiomyopathy.*
Congestive heart failure (CHF). See *Heart failure, congestive.*
Constrictive pericarditis. See *Pericarditis.*
Contraceptives, oral, 70
Convulsions, 148
Coronary arteries, 77t, 126
Coronary artery disease, 75-82
  men and, 78
  pacemakers and, 141
  point of maximal impulse and, 48
  risk factors, 76, 78
  S_4 and, 52
  women and, 78
Coronary artery perfusion, 105, 107, 137
Coronary bypass graft, 111-112
Coronary ventriculography, 64t
Cor pulmonale, acute, 137
Corrigan's pulse, 17t
CPK (creatine phosphokinase), 88t
Crepitant rales, 98
Cushing's syndrome, 72t
Cyanosis
  cardiac tamponade and, 144
  central, 28t, 46
  heart defects and, 28t
  in child, 15-16
  peripheral, 28t, 46
  tetralogy of Fallot and, 31
  vascular disease and, 161t

D
Death. See *Mortality.*
Declamping hypotension phenomenon, 167
Dehydration, 47
Dentistry, 117, 120
Depression, 91-92
Dermatitis, stasis, 161
Diabetes, 76t
Diabetic neuropathy, 156

Diagnostic tests, 55-66
  common, 61t
Diastole, 20, 22, 50-54
Diastolic gallop, 98
Diet, 76, 76t, 89t
Dissecting aneurysm, 167t
Distal phalangeal depth (DPD), 46, 46t
Dressler syndrome, 121. See also *Postmyocardial infarction.*
Dyskinesis, 64, 85t
Dyspnea, 70, 94, 131
  in children, 16
  pneumothorax and, 38
  pulmonary edema and, 98

E
Echocardiography, 57-58
  endocarditis and, 117
  rheumatic heart disease and, 124
  ventricular aneurysm and, 111
Echophonocardiography, 58
Edema, 161-162
  ankle, 93
  dependent, 94
  hypertension and, 70
  in children, 16
  pulmonary. See *Pulmonary edema.*
  right heart failure and, 30t
  skin evaluation and, 47
  X-rays and, 56
EKG. See *Electrocardiogram.*
Elderly, 94, 117, 155, 156
Electrocardiogram, 58-60
  acute myocardial infarction and, 85-86, 87t
  ambulatory, 129
  cardiomyopathy and, 130
  reading, 60t
  stress test and, 59-60
  12-lead, 58t
  waves of, 59t
Electrodes, 144
Embolectomy, 140
Embolism, 133-140, 134t
  amniotic fluid, 134t
  chest surgery and, 144
  endocardial pathogens and, 117
  endocarditis and, 118t
  fat, 134t
  pulmonary, 46. See also *Pulmonary embolism.*
  thrombus, 134t
  tumor, 134t

ventricular aneurysm and, 111-112
Endocarditis, 118, 118t, 119
  antibiotics, high-risk patients and, 120
  bacterial, 116-121
  infection and, 148
  rheumatic heart disease and, 123
Exercise, 78, 94
  angina and, 82
  ASO and, 158-159
  pacemakers and, 148
  venous stasis and, 136
Eyes, 39-40

F
False aneurysm, 167t
Familial tendencies, 70, 78
Fat embolism, 134t
Fetal circulation, 23-24, 25t
Fever, 17t, 117, 117t
Fibrinous pericarditis. See Pericarditis.
Fibrosis, 149
Fluids and electrolytes, 39, 40
Fluoroscopy, 57-58
Fungi, 115-116
Fusiform aneurysm, 166t

G
Gallop rhythm, 20, 116
Gangrene, 161t
Glomerulonephritis, 72t

H
Hammon's sign, 20, 22
Headache, 68, 71
Heart, 20t, 48t, 49
  enlarged, 55, 56
  child, 18-22
  normal pressures and O_2 saturation, 52t
  pacemakers and, 142
  rate, 68
    pacemaker failure and, 144, 148
  rhythm, abnormal, 19-20, 85t
Heart block, 19, 148, 150
Heart chamber wall, 64
Heart defects, congenital, 23-32, 28t, 46
Heart disease, 17t, 115-124
  congenital, 15, 116-117
  congestive, 93-94
  hypertension and, 71
  organic, 20

Heart, enlarged. See Cardiomegaly.
Heart failure, 30t, 38, 94
  acute myocardial infarction and, 86, 89
  cardiogenic shock and, 111
  cardiomyopathy and, 126
  children and, 15, 32
  congestive, 93-102, 95t, 131
    atrial septal defects and, 29
    cyanosis and, 46
    IHSS and, 130
    jaundice and, 46
    left-sided, 94
    myocardial infarction and, 89
    myocarditis and, 116
    patent ductus arteriosus and, 29
    pleural effusion and, 96t
  elderly and, 94
  pulmonary edema and, 89
  venous distention and, 46
Heart murmurs, 53-54, 123
Heart muscle disease. See Cardiomyopathy.
Heart, rupture of, 89
Heart sounds, 20, 22, 49-54, 51t
  acute myocardial infarction and, 84-85
  normal, 19
  S_1, 50
  S_2, 50, 52
  S_3, 52
  S_4, 52-53
Heart valves, 49-54, 116
Hemochromatosis, 126
Hemoglobin, 23-24
Hemorrhage, 106t
Heparin administration, 140t
Hepatojugular reflex, 94
Hepatomegaly, 93-94
Heredity. See Familial tendencies.
Hiccups, 144, 149
High density lipoproteins (HDL). See Lipoproteins, high density.
Holter monitor, 129
Hospitalization, child, 34, 38t
Hypercoagulability, 134
Hyperkalemia, 39
Hyperlipidemia, 76, 78, 160t
Hypertension, 67-74, 68t
  arterial, 19, 20
  biofeedback and, 73
  cardiogenic shock and, 103-104

congestive heart failure and, 94
coronary artery disease and, 76t
ejaculation failure and, 73
essential, 69, 70, 71
in blacks, 68, 70
malignant, 70-71
point of maximal impulse and, 48
pulmonary, 22, 137
retinopathy and, 71
S_4 and, 52
secondary, 69, 72t
statistics, 67-68
stress and, 70
Hypertensive crisis, 71t
Hyperthyroidism, 17t, 20, 128
Hyperventilation, 98
Hypocalcemia, 39
Hypokalemia, 39
Hypokinesis, 64, 85t
Hypotension, 104, 107
  cardiac catheterization and, 62
  declamping phenomenon, 167
  pulmonary obstruction and, 137
Hypovolemia, 39, 105-106
Hypoxemia, 104
Hypoxia, 46, 98, 104

I
Idiopathic hypertrophic subaortic stenosis (IHSS). See Cardiomyopathy, hypertrophic.
Immobilization. See Patient, immobilized.
Infants, 16, 30t. See also Children.
Infections, 115-124
  ASO and, 158
  endocarditis and, 116-117
    prevention of, 119-120
  myocarditis and, 115-116
  pacemakers and, 148
  pericarditis and, 121
Inotropic agents, 132
Inspection, 46-47
Intensive care unit (ICU), 40
Interphalangeal depth (IPD), 46, 46t
Interventricular septum, rupture of, 90
Intra-aortic balloon pump (IABP), 106t-107t, 107-111. See also Swan-Ganz catheter.
  position of, 109t
  weaning, 108, 108t
Intracardiac shunt, 29

Ischemia, 141, 156, 161t
Ischemic myocardium. See
     Myocardial ischemia.

J
Jaundice, 46
Judkins technique, 64, 66
Jugular vein, 46, 47

K
Kidneys, 70-71, 104
Kwashiorkor, 128

L
Lactic acidosis. See *Metabolic
     acidosis.*
LDH (lactic dehydrogenase), 88t
Left anterior descending artery
     (LAD), 77t
Left border of cardiac dullness
     (LBCD), 49
Left circumflex artery (LCF), 77t
Left ventricular end-diastolic
     pressure (LVEDP), 104t, 105
Leg pain, 155-162
Lipoproteins, high density, 81t
Liver, enlarged. See
     Hepatomegaly.
Lumbar pain, 164
Lung cancer, 46, 46t
Lung disease, chronic
     obstructive, 46
Lung scans, 139t
Lungs, 98t

M
Marfan's syndrome, 18
Medical history, 45
Membrane oxygenator, 39
Metabolic acidosis, 98, 102, 104,
     107
Midclavicular line (MCL), 49
Mitral regurgitation,54, 123t
     acute myocardial infarction
         and, 84
     coarctation of aorta and, 30
     endocarditis and, 117, 117t
     myocarditis and, 116
     rheumatic heart disease and,
         123
Mitral stenosis, 19, 22, 54, 123t
     rhematic heart disease and,
         123-124
Mitral valve, 22, 50, 62
     endocarditis and, 117
     hypertrophic cardiomyopathy
         and, 131

Starr Edwards prosthesis, 120t
Monitoring, 132
Mortality, 15, 111
Murmurs. See *Heart murmurs.*
Myocardial disease, primary. See
     Cardiomyopathy.
Myocardial function, 62, 64
Myocardial hypertrophy, 57
Myocardial hypertrophy,
     idiopathic. See
     Cardiomyopathy.
Myocardial imaging, 60-61
Myocardial infarction, 83-92
     cardiogenic shock and,
         103-111
     congestive heart failure and, 94
     diet, 89t
     emotional problems of, 90-92
     enzyme levels in, 88t
     pacemakers and, 141
     pain and, 53t, 80, 122
     pericarditis and, 121
     S$_4$ and, 52
     stress testing and, 59
     treatment goals, 90t-91t
     type A personality and, 82t
     ventricular rupture and, 112
     wall motion and, 64
Myocardial ischemia, 30, 79, 105,
     149
Myocardial necrosis, 86
Myocardial perfusion, 131
Myocardiopathy. See
     Cardiomyopathy.
Myocarditis, 115-116, 116t
     cardiomyopathy and, 128
     rheumatic heart disease and,
         123

N
Neck pulsation, 46
Neck vein distention, 94, 144
Neonates. See *Children.*
Nephrosclerosis, 70
Nervous system, autonomic, 69
Neurologic assessment, 39-40
Neurological disorders, 126
Neuropathy, 156
Newborn, 23-32
Nicotine, 73
Nocturia, 70, 93

O
Obesity, 70, 78
Oliguria, 104
Optic fundi, 71
Orthopnea, 16, 70, 94, 98, 131

Osler's nodes, 117, 117t
Osteoarthritis, 156
Oxygen saturation, 23-24, 52t
Oxygen therapy, 101t

P
Pacemakers, artificial, 141-150
     capturing, 149
     competition, 150
     firing, 149
     infection and, 148
     malfunctions in, 144, 148-150
     monitoring, 148-149
     patient tips, 148t
     questions patients ask, 147t
     sensing, 149-150
     temporary, 142, 148
     transvenous, 145t
     types of, 146t
Pain, 53t, 105, 112, 117t
Palpation, 21t, 47-49
Papillary muscle rupture, 90
Papilledema, 70-71
Paradoxical pulse, 47-48
Parents, support of, 33-34
Paroxysmal nocturnal dyspnea.
     See *Dyspnea.*
Patent ductus arteriosus (PDA),
     26t, 29-30
     blood pressure and, 19t
     pulmonary ejection click and,
         22
     pulse pressure and, 17t
Patient assessment, 45-54
Patient, examination of, 49-54
     child, 18-22
Patient, immobilized, 133, 136
Patient teaching, 72-73
     acute myocardial infarction
         and, 92
     children and, 35
     coronary artery disease and,
         75-76
     pacemakers and, 143, 144, 150
     pulmonary embolism and, 140
Percussion, 49
Pericardial effusions, 57, 122
Pericardial friction rub, 54, 90,
     122
     in children, 20
Pericardial tap, 122
Pericardiectomy, 122
Pericardiocentesis, 112, 114
Pericarditis, 121-122, 122t
     acute myocardial infarction
         and, 90
     constrictive, 48, 121

fibrinous, 121
friction rub and, 54
pain of, 53t, 80
rheumatic heart disease and, 123
Peripheral vascular resistance, 68-69
Petechiae, 117, 117t
Pharyngitis, acute, 123
Pheochromocytoma, 70, 72t, 128
Phlebography, 159
Phlebotomy, 102
Phonocardiography, 58
Plateau pulse. See *Pulsus torlus.*
Pleural effusion, 96t
Pleural rub, 20
Pleuro-pericardial window, 122
Pneumonia, 144
Pneumothorax, 38-39
Pneumothorax, tension, 38
Point of maximal impulse (PMI), 48
Polyarthritis, 123
Polycythemia, 16
Postmyocardial infarction, 90
Postoperative care, 37t, 39
monitoring patient, 36, 38
of aneurysm patient, 166-167
of chest tubes, 114
of children, 40
pacemaker implantation and, 143-150
Potassium loss, 73
Precordial bulge, 85
Preload. See *Ventricular filling pressure.*
Premature ventricular contractions (PVCs), 39, 148
Preoperative care, 33, 35-36, 166
Protozoas, 115
Public Health Service report, 136
Pulmonary artery catheter, 166
Pulmonary artery pressure, 104t, 106
Pulmonary congestion, 55
Pulmonary edema, 97-102, 100t
acute myocardial infarction and, 89
alveolar stage, 98
bronchial stage, 98-100
congestive heart failure and, 93, 97-102
effect on lungs, 94
interstitial stage, 98
nursing management of, 99t
Pulmonary ejection click, 22
Pulmonary embolism, 133-140,

138t. See also *Embolism.*
acute cor pulmonale and, 137
acute myocardial infarction and, 89
heparin administration in, 140t
pulmonary infarction and, 137
Pulmonary hypertension, 137
Pulmonary hypertension, chronic, 55-56
Pulmonary infarction, 137
Pulmonary rales, 94, 98
Pulmonary stenosis, 30-31
Pulmonary venous pressure, 131
Pulmonary wedge pressure, 104t
Pulmonic regurgitation, 54
Pulmonic stenosis, 54
Pulse, 17t, 48
ASO and, 156
in child, 16, 19
peripheral, 47, 49t
pressure, 17t, 19t
rate, 17t, 144
in children, 18t
pacemaker and, 148-149
Pulsus alternans, 17t, 47
Pulsus bigeminus, 17t
Pulsus bisferiens, 17t, 130
Pulsus paradoxus, 17t, 38
Pulsus torlus, 17t
PVCs. See *Ventricular contractions, premature.*

Q
Quadruple rhythm, 53

R
Radioisotopic myocardial imaging, 111
Radiology, 55-57, 130
Raynaud's disease, 161t
Raynaud's phenomenon, 161t
Renal hypertension, 72t
Renal ischemia, 69
Renal parenchymal disease, 70
Renal vascular stenosis, 70
Renin-angiotensin system, 104
Respiration, 16t, 102
assessment of child and, 15
cyanosis, children and, 16
pulmonary edema and, 98, 100
signs of distress, 38
Respiratory care, 38-39
aneurysm surgery and, 167-168
Respiratory infections, 16, 32
Retinopathy, 71
Rheumatic fever, 122-123
children and, 15, 123

heart rhythm and, 20
myocarditis and, 116
pulse rate and, 17t
Rheumatic heart disease, 122-124
endocarditis and, 116-117
myocarditis and, 116t
Rheumatic mitral regurgitant murmur, 85
Rheumatic myocarditis, 126
Rheumatic valvular disease, 94, 126
Rheumatoid arthritis, 121
Rotating tourniquets, 102

S
S_1, 50
S_2, 50, 52
S_3, 52
S_4, 52-53
Saccular aneurysm, 166t
Sarcoidosis, 126
Sclerosing agents, 161
Semilunar valvular stenosis, 52
Septicemia, 148
Sexuality, 79, 82, 92
SGOT (serum glutamic-oxaloacetic transaminase), 88t
Sinus arrhythmia, 20
Sinus tachycardia, 106
Skin, 15, 46, 47, 156, 157t
Smoking, 75, 76, 78, 158
Sodium, 73
Sones technique, 64
Spider veins. See *Telangiectases.*
Splenomegaly, 117
Splinter hemorrhages, 117, 117t
Squatting, 31-32
Starling curve, 167
Starr Edwards mitral valve, 120t
Sternal angle, 47t
Sternotomy, 112, 114
Stokes-Adams attack, 142t
Stress, 76, 78, 90-91
hypertension and, 70
biofeedback and, 73
Stress testing, 59-60
Subacute bacterial endocarditis (SBE). See *Endocarditis, bacterial.*
Summation gallop, 53, 81
Support stockings, 161-162
Surgery, 39-40, 144, 148
abdominal aneurysm and, 164, 166-167

arterial occlusion and, 158
cardiogenic shock and, 108
children and, 33-40, 35t
coronary arteriography and, 64
hypertrophic cardiomyopathy
    and, 131
jaundice and, 46
open-heart, 112, 117
pacemakers and, 141, 144, 148
pneumothorax and, 38
rheumatic heart disease and,
    124
septal defects and, 28, 29
stress test and, 59
tetralogy of Fallot and, 32
valvular damage and, 120
varicose veins and, 159
venous stasis and, 135-136
Swan-Ganz catheter, 104t, 132
    complications, 106t-107t
Swan-Ganz thermodilution
    catheter, 105t
Sympatholytics, 72
Syncope, 148
Systemic hypotension, 137
Systemic lupus erythematosus
    (SLE), 121
Systole, 20, 50-54
    ventricular, 48, 54
Systolic ejection murmur, 130
Systolic murmurs, 84, 116, 117,
    117t

T
Tachyarrhythmias, 142
Tachycardia, 17t, 104, 116
    ventricular, 148, 149
Tachypnea, 16, 30t, 94
Tamponade, cardiac, 112, 114
    paradoxical pulse and, 48
    venous distention and, 46
    restlessness and, 144

Telangiectasies, 161
Tetralogy of Fallot, 27t, 30-32
    signs of, 16
Thoracentesis, 38, 96t
Thoracotomy, 38
Thromboangiitis obliterans. See
    Buerger's disease.
Thrombocytopenia, 106t
Thromboembolism, 134t
Thrombophlebitis, 148, 159, 162
Thrombus formation, 134-135
    mural, 111
    Swan-Ganz catheter and, 106t
Thyrotoxicosis, 20, 22
Toxemia, 70
Transmural infarction, 89
Transposition of great vessels,
    27t, 32
Tricuspid regurgitation, 54
Tricuspid valve, 22, 50, 54
Tumor emboli, 134t
Tumors, atrial, 22
Type A personality, 82t

U
Ulcers, stasis, 161, 162t
Ultrasound. See
    Echocardiography.
Unna boot bandage, 162t
Urine output, 104, 144

V
Valsalva maneuver, 136
Valsalva, sinuses of, 64
Valves, 123-124
    echocardiography and, 57
    endocarditis and, 117
    prosthetic, 120, 120t
Valvular regurgitation, 52
Valvular stenosis, 46, 62
Varicose veins, 158t, 159-162
Vascular disease, 161t, 155-162

leg pains and, 155
Vasopressors, 104, 107
Venae cavae, 52t
Venous distention, 46, 47, 47t
Venous hum, 22
Venous insufficiency, 159-162
Venous pressure, increased, 144
Venous stasis, 135, 136, 136t,
    137t, 160t
Ventilation, mechanical, 38
Ventricles, 52t
Ventricular aneurysm. See
    Aneurysm, ventricular.
Ventricular diastole, 54
Ventricular dilatation, 116
Ventricular extrasystoles, 148
Ventricular failure, 47, 52, 97
Ventricular fibrillation, 108, 149,
    150
Ventricular filling pressure, 84t
Ventricular gallop, 49, 52, 81, 84
Ventricular hypertrophy, 30, 31,
    49
Ventricular myotomy, 131
Ventricular outflow obstruction, 30
Ventricular septal defect (VSD),
    24, 26t, 28, 62
    pulmonary ejection click and,
    22
    tetralogy of Fallot and, 30-31
Ventriculography, 64, 111
Virchow, Rudolf, 160t
Viruses, 115, 116t, 128

W
Water-hammer pulse. See
    Corrigan's pulse.
Weight gain, 94
Women, 78

X
X-ray. See *Radiology.*

SUGGESTED FURTHER READING

Alpert, Joseph S., and Gary S. Francis. MANUAL OF CORONARY CARE. Boston, Little, Brown and Company, 1977.

Andreoli, Kathleen G. COMPREHENSIVE CARDIAC CARE: A TEXT FOR NURSES AND OTHER HEALTH PROFESSIONALS. St. Louis, C. V. Mosby Company, 1975.

Armington, Sister Catherine, and Helen Creighton. NURSING OF PEOPLE WITH CARDIOVASCULAR PROBLEMS. Boston, Little, Brown and Company, 1971.

Bates, Barbara. A GUIDE TO PHYSICAL EXAMINATION. Philadelphia, J. B. Lippincott Company, 1974.

Ellestad, Myrvin H. STRESS TESTING: PRINCIPLES AND PRACTICE. Philadelphia, F. A. Davis Company, 1975.

Fowler, Noble O. EXAMINATION OF THE HEART: INSPECTION AND PALPATION OF VENOUS AND ARTERIAL PULSES, PART 2. New York, American Heart Association, 1972.

Harvey, A. McGehee, et. al., eds. THE PRINCIPLES AND PRACTICE OF MEDICINE. New York, Appleton-Century-Crofts, 1976.

Hurst, J. Willis, et. al., eds. THE HEART. New York, McGraw-Hill Book Company, 1974.

Hurst, J. Willis, and Robert C. Schlant. EXAMINATION OF THE HEART: INSPECTION AND PALPATION OF THE ANTERIOR CHEST, PART 3. New York, American Heart Association, 1972.

Keele, Cyril A., and Eric Niel, eds. SAMSON WRIGHT'S APPLIED PHYSIOLOGY. London, Oxford University Press, 1971.

Kernicki, Jeanette, et. al. CARDIOVASCULAR NURSING: RATIONALE FOR THERAPY AND NURSING APPROACH. New York, G. P. Putnam's Sons, 1971.

King, Ouida M. CARE OF THE CARDIAC SURGICAL PATIENT. St. Louis, C. V. Mosby Company, 1975.

Lowell, J. R. PLEURAL EFFUSIONS: A COMPREHENSIVE TREATISE. Baltimore, University Park Press, 1976.

Markowitz, Milton, and Leon Gordis. RHEUMATIC FEVER. Philadelphia, W. B. Saunders Company, 1972.

Meltzer, L.E., et. al. CONCEPTS AND PRACTICES OF INTENSIVE CARE FOR NURSE SPECIALISTS. Maryland, The Charles Press Publishers, Inc., 1976.

Meltzer, L. E. et al. INTENSIVE CORONARY CARE: A MANUAL FOR NURSES. Maryland, The Charles Press Publishers, Inc., 1977.

Modell, Walter, et al. HANDBOOK OF CARDIOLOGY FOR NURSES. New York, Springer Publishing Company, Inc., 1966.

Ravin, Abe, et al. AUSCULTATION OF THE HEART. Chicago, Year Book Medical Publishers, 1977.

Russek, H. F., and B. L. Zohman. CARDIOVASCULAR THERAPY. New York, Robert E. Krieger Publishing Company, 1971.

Sabiston, David C., ed. DAVIS-CHRISTOPHER TEXTBOOK OF SURGERY. Philadelphia, W. B. Saunders Company, 1977.

Sanderson, R. G. THE CARDIAC PATIENT: A COMPREHENSIVE APPROACH. Philadelphia, W. B. Saunders Company, 1972.

Scipien, Gladys, et. al. COMPREHENSIVE PEDIATRIC NURSING. New York, McGraw-Hill Book Company, 1975.

Selzer, Arthur. PRINCIPLES OF CLINICAL CARDIOLOGY. Philadelphia. W. B. Saunders Company, 1975.

Sweetwood, Hannelore. THE PATIENT IN THE CORONARY CARE UNIT. New York, Springer Publishing Company, Inc., 1976.

Tucker, Susan, et. al. PATIENT CARE STANDARDS. St. Louis, C. V. Mosby Company, 1975.

Vaughn, Victor, and R. James McKay, eds. NELSON TEXTBOOK OF PEDIATRICS. Philadelphia, W. B. Saunders Company, 1975.

Waechter, Eugenia, and Florence Blake. NURSING CARE OF CHILDREN. Philadelphia, J. B. Lippincott Company, 1976.

ACKNOWLEDGEMENTS

p. 18   Table and statistical information courtesy: Vaughan and McKay, *Textbook of Pediatrics*, Tenth edition. W. B. Saunders Company, 1975, p. 1003, 1098.

p. 29   Photos courtesy: *The Heart*, Fourth edition by Hurst et. al. Copyright 1978 by McGraw-Hill, Inc. Used with permission of McGraw-Hill Book Company.

p. 37   Photos courtesy: Public Relations Department, Children's Hospital of Philadelphia.

p. 57   X-ray courtesy: Peter G. Lavine, MD, Crozer-Chester Medical Center, Chester, Pa.

p. 64   Cines courtesy: Peter G. Lavine, MD.

p. 70   Photo courtesy: Temple University Department of Ophthalmology, Philadelphia, Pa.

p. 79   Cine courtesy: Peter G. Lavine, MD.

p. 96   X-ray courtesy: Peter G. Lavine, MD.

p. 111   Cine courtesy: Peter G. Lavine, MD.

p. 117   Photo courtesy: Gerald Pearlman, Skin and Cancer Hospital, Temple University Health Sciences Center, Philadelphia, Pa.

p. 120   X-ray courtesy: Peter G. Lavine, MD.

p. 129   Photos courtesy: Medical Monitors, Wyncote, Pa.

p. 139   Scans courtesy: John Reilley, Temple University Hospital, Department of Nuclear Medicine, Philadelphia, Pa.

p. 161   Photos courtesy: Moschella and Pillsbury, *Dermatology*. W. B. Saunders Company, 1975. Volume 1, p. 841.

p. 177   Rehab chart courtesy: Kathryn A. Hoffman, MD, Assistant Professor Rehabilitation Medicine, Emory University, Atlanta, Georgia.